PREDICTING EXCELLENCE IN FIELD HOCKEY

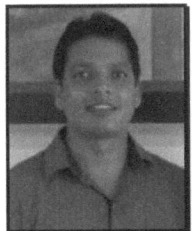

Dr. Sanjay Kumar Prajapati

FIRST EDITION

LAXMI BOOK PUBLICATION
258/34, Raviwar Peth,
Solapur-413005
Cell: +91 9595359435

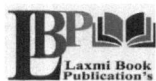

Rs: 250 /-

PREDICTING EXCELLENCE IN FIELD HOCKEY
Dr. Sanjay Kumar Prajapati

© 2015 by Laxmi Book Publication, Solapur

ISBN- 978-1-329-13830-8

Published by,

Laxmi Book Publication,
258/34, Raviwar Peth,
Solapur, Maharashtra, India.

Contact No. : +91 9595 359 435
Website: http://www.isrj.org
Email ID: ayisrj@yahoo.in

ACKNOWLEDGEMENT

At the very outset, I wish to express the most sincere gratitude to my supervisor, Prof. Sushma Ghildyal, Department of Physical Education, Faculty of Arts, Banaras Hindu University, Varanasi for suggesting me the problem, her keen interest, invaluable help, continuous encouragement, her untiring patience, constructive criticism and constant motivation during entire research work that enabled me to reach at this stage of completion. Whenever, I fumbled in darkness of confusion and dilemma, her suggestions, criticism and guidance enlighten my path for clearing the horizons. Apart from thesis matters, his interests in leading a healthy and disciplined life also influenced me.

I am grateful to Prof. D. K Dureha, Head, Department of Physical Education, Banaras Hindu University, Varanasi, for his perpetual inspiration and inimitable teaching as a source of infinite acumen. He has always been a source of encouragement for me during my entire work.

A deep sense of gratitude is expressed to Prof. B.C Kapri, Dr. Rajeev Chaudhary, Dr. Abhimanyu Singh, Dr. Akhil Mehrotra, Dr. Vikram Singh and Dr. T. Onima Readdy, Assistant professor, Department of Physical Education, Banaras Hindu University, Varanasi for being a constant source of inspiration and for their able guidance and suggestions.

Research Scholar expresses his deep gratitude and respect to Dr. Rajeev Vyas, Assistant professor, Department of Physical Education, Banaras Hindu University, Varanasi, for his valuable suggestions on various aspects of this study. I am also thankful to sir for being my source of inspiration.

Research Scholar expresses his gratitude thanks to his friends Dayanand Singh, Anil Yadav, Abhishek Verma, Shailesh Kumar, Sourabh Singh for their deep and honest cooperation in data collection and also for motivating and for developing faith in myself, as without help of these people, data collection and initiation of this study was not possible.

I extend my sincere thanks to Principal of Guru Govind Singh Sports College Lucknow and Regional Director of sports Bhopal SAI and all the coaches Paramjeet Singh, Hockey Coach Ranjeet Raj, Hockey Coach Karan Singh Thapa, Hockey Coach Raju Sonkar, Hockey Coach, Organizers and specially the players who acted as Subject and helped me during data collection and extending all the help during measurements and other necessary help for collecting the study material. Their enthusiasm & cooperation is priceless, and without their support I would not been able to finish my work.

I extend my grateful thank to my senior Dr. Rajive Partap Singh Dr. Ashish Singh, Dr. Rajnish Chand Tirpathi Sir Dr. Devpal Rana, Anoop Kumar Singh, Chandrabhan Singh, Dr. Manas Sah, Shyam Lal Yadav for their suggestions and motivation.

I am also thankful to Vivek Tiwari, Sandeep Singh, Vikash Yadav, Abhinav Singh, Linet Khakha, Neha Arora, Pravesh Dubey, Shazia Rashidi, Deepak Dhaka, Richa Singh, Rahul Singh, Asif Kaleem, Satyajeet and all the research scholars of the department who helped me openhandedly.

I am indebted to my Father Sh. Shyam Bihari Prajapati and my Mother Smt. Shanti Devi, Sister Archana Prajapati, Brother

Anand Prajapati and Manoj Prajapati for their moral support and encouragement. They were the source of inspiration for me during my research work.

I would like to thanks my friends Mr. Ashwani Kumar, Mr Sujeet Singh, Amit Singh, Mukti singh Srinet, Bheeshm Singh whose cooperation and motivation helped me to carry out my research work successfully.

I am grateful to all the Students of Department. They were like family members to me and helped me whenever I asked, and without their cooperation and priceless help this work would have not seen the ray of hope towards the completion of this thesis.

I will fail in duty if I will not recognize the sincere support of office employees of department, Mr. Alok, Mr. Pankaj and Gautam ji. These are the pillars and without their humble support, smooth completion of the study was not possible.

Lastly, my warm appreciation and thanks for all those, who had been the constant source of inspiration either directly or indirectly.

Dr. Sanjay Kumar Prajapati

PREFACE

In recent scenario growth of a country, institution or profession depends on quality of research done in particular area. Our climate, atmosphere, geographical conditions and culture play a important role in the psychological and physiological characteristics of population and sports persons also. It has been well establish fact that research made development of new techniques, facilities and human friendly atmosphere. While it has also develop the idea about better health which deals with way of thinking, life style, involvement in sports and physical activity which lead us to a healthy life.

A sincere effort has been made by the scholar to understand the effect of environment and geographical conditions on sport person and their performance. In this respect the first chapter of the study is the introductory part that gives an over view of the purpose of the study. This chapter includes delimitations of the study that describes the frame work of the study. In the limitations of this study several factors are described which were beyond the control of the investigator that might have affected the study. The chapter also describes and explains various technical terms which may not be easier to understand by common man.

The second chapter includes review of the related literature that the scholar has gathered through various sources such as libraries and internet.

The third chapter procedure comprises of selection of subjects, selection of variables, Criterion measures, collection of data, administration of Test and statistical techniques used for analysis of data.

The fourth chapter of the study includes analysis of data and the result of the study. These are presented in the form of findings, discussion of findings. The findings of the study have been presented in tabular form in this chapter.

In the fifth and the concluding chapter a brief summary of the total work is written. This chapter also deals with the conclusions made from the results lastly; recommendations are given by the scholar points wise for future researches.

Dr. Sanjay Kumar Prajapati

CONTENT

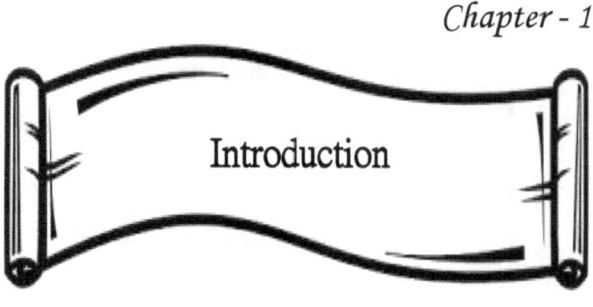

Chapter - 1

Introduction

"One man practicing sportsmanship is far better than fifty preaching it."

-Knute Rockne

Movement and activity are basic functions needed by human organism to grow, develop, and maintain health. However, physical activity is no longer a natural part of our existence. We live in an automated world where most of the activities that used to require strenuous physical exertion, can be accomplished by machines with the simple pull of a handle or push of a button. For instance, if there is a need to go to a store most of the people drive their automobiles. Similarly, during a normal visit to a multi-level shopping mall, it can easily be observed that almost everyone chooses to ride the escalators instead of taking the stairs. Automobiles, elevators, escalators, telephone, intercoms, remote controls, electric garage door openers, etc. are all modern-day commodities that minimize the amount of movement and efforts required by the human body.

By nature, human beings are competitive and ambitious for the excellence in all athletic performances. Not only every man but every nation wants to show their supremacy by challenging other Individual, state, group or nation. This challenge stimulates, inspires and motivates the entire nation to strive for faster, higher, and further. It compels to exaggerate, strength, endurance and skills in the present competitive sports world.

The sports world comprises not only of winning and losing but also of playing a game. With positive attitude today, the emphasis is on excelling in whatever one does, whether one is on the field playing or one is training the players; both have a very responsible and important role to perform.

Games and sports have been prominent in Man's heritage, traced back to his earliest consciousness they are included in his cultural perspective and have complemented the search for understanding and meaning in life.

Sports provide an outlet for the suppressed internal feeling of an individual. It is like a safety valve to 'blow off the steam'. Nervous, tired and frustrated person can take sports as a tonic. Sports can be utilized for students to dissociate them from the monotony of books and the pressure of studies. Sports further provide a learning situation in formal and informal ways in which the participants learn to modify certain qualities in a unique way. Sport activity is determined by four sub-systems, i.e. the cultural, social, personal and organic systems. Sports also play a vital role in development of the individual's character and desirable personality traits which is important to survive in human society. There are several categories of sports according to the aim, objective and organizational point of view. There are sprint sports, endurance sports, power sports, technical sports, tactical sports, water sports, precision sports etc, which might be individual or team sports or measurable and non measurable sports. Hockey is one of the team sports which demands high level technical and tactical abilities along with desired level of Fitness.

Field hockey is played on gravel, natural grass, sand-based or water-based artificial turf, with a small, hard ball. The game is popular among both males and females in many parts of the world, particularly in Europe, Asia, Australia, New Zealand and South Africa. In most countries, the game is played between single-sex sides, although they can be mixed-sex.

The governing body is the 116-member International Hockey Federation (FIH). Men's field hockey has been played at each summer Olympic Games since 1908 (except 1912 and 1924), while women's field hockey has been played at the Summer Olympic Games since 1980.

Field hockey is a team sport in which a team of players attempt to score goals by hitting, pushing or flicking the ball with hockey sticks into the opposing team's goal. Its official name is simply hockey, and this is the common name for it in many countries. However, the name field hockey is used in countries where the word hockey is usually reserved for another form of hockey, such as ice hockey or street hockey.

Amongst most of the sports that is being played these days Hockey is one of the favourite of all. In the general sense it is a kind of sport in which two teams compete by trying to makeover the ball into the opponent's nest using a hockey stick.

However, games like hockey have been played in almost every populated region in the globe from Ancient Greece to North America. Hockey has also been played in the ancient times in both foot and in horseback. This type of hockey is played on gravel or natural grass with a small hard ball.

Nowadays it is played on a special type of artificial surface known as the Astroturf. The body composition and energy turnover are highly inter-related and closely linked with the functional capacity of the organism. Therefore evaluation of one's body composition is useful for understanding the functional aspect of the sportsman. The use of this science is immense utility in so far as sportsmen are concerned. Moreover, the incidence of beginning age obesity is increasing considerably in industrialized countries and affluent classes in many other countries. The cause of obesity is the way of the life. Further in participation of exercise of game the obese proves less active.

Modern field hockey sticks are J-shaped and constructed of a composite of wood, glass fibre or carbon fibre (sometimes both) and have a curved hook at the playing end, a flat surface on the playing side and curved surface on the rear side. While current field hockey appeared in the mid-18th century in England, primarily in schools, it was not until the first half of the 19th century that it became firmly established. The first club was created in 1849 at Blackheath in south-east London. Field hockey is the national sport of India and Pakistan.

According to nature, hockey is entirely different from many team games. Hockey is a game of grace and beauty which is based on technical skill, which require years of practice for being mastered in particular skill, which requires more and more concentration and patience with higher degree of fitness. Along with fitness and year of practice another factor which affects the performance is physique of players because it is well known fact that physique plays a dominating role in performance of player.

Hockey has several regular international tournaments for both men and women. These include the Olympic Games, the quadrennial Hockey World Cups, the annual Champions Trophies and World Cups for juniors.

The International Hockey Federation (FIH) is the global governing body. It organizes events such as the Hockey World Cup and Women's Hockey World Cup. The Hockey Rules Board under FIH produces rules for the sport.

Many countries have extensive club competitions for junior and senior players. Despite the large number of participants, hockey is thought to be the field team sport with the second largest number of participants worldwide (the first being association football), club hockey is not a large spectator sport and few players play as full-time professionals.

In countries where winter prevents play outdoors, hockey is played indoors during the off-season. This variant, indoor field Hockey differs in a number of respects. For example, it is 6-a-side rather than 11, the field is reduced to approximately 40 m x 20 m; the shooting circles are 9m; players may not raise the ball outside the circle nor hit it. The sidelines are replaced with barriers to rebound the ball.

Field hockey is an intermittent endurance sport involving short sprinting as well as movement with and without ball (Manna et al., 2009). Successful performance in field hockey is influenced by physiological and anthropometric characteristics such as body size and composition, functional parameters (physical capacity) (Scott, 1991; Singh et al., 2010) and fitness (strength, speed, anaerobic and aerobic capacity, agility) (Nikitushkin & Guba, 1998). In field hockey, players are to bend forward to the ground for the maximum groundwork and to cover a wider range all around during the game (Sodhi, 1991) and maximum strain comes over the back muscles as well as abdominal muscles during the entire duration of the game. Estimation of back strength of Indian inter-university male hockey players and significant positive correlations of back strength with height, weight, BMI, hip circumference, % lean body mass and abdominal muscle endurance was reported (Koley et al., 2012). Evaluation of anthropometric, physiological and skill-related tests for talent identification in female field hockey was also reported (Keogh et al., 2003). Anthropometric characteristics and physiological variables were compared too, among the national hockey players of India, Pakistan and Sri Lanka (Singh et al., 2010). Hockey players playing in different positions found to differ on some anthropometric measurements and body composition (Karkare, 2011).

Field hockey is a team sport with heavy demands on the player's physiology. As a consequence, elite players show a high degree of leanness. Furthermore, team mean percentage body fat was found to bear a relation with finishing position in a sample of 12 teams playing the South African Senior Provincial tournament. On the contrary, in Australia, sub elite male field hockey players did not differ from Senior or Youth select sides in mass, height, or body fat levels. Elite level sport tends to self-select individuals with morphological characteristics which respond optimally to its physical demands. Since field hockey requires players to spend time in a crouched position, having long arms may be an advantage in this activity. Data on 33 male field hockey players from the Montreal

5

Olympic Games showed them to have proportionally longer arm and fore arm lengths when compared to a reference Canadian university student sample. Scott did not find any correlation between functional arm length and playing ability in his large sample of players.

Human performance is a composition of many variables such as structure of the body, the specific measurements of the limbs, circumferences, breadth and body build. Since motor performance is an outcome of various variables, there may be a direct relationship between certain specific measurements and motor performance. The type of individual's structure is an essential factor in his motor performance than a normal person.

Physiology is the science of functioning of all the organs and systems of an organism. For the physiological system of the body to be fit, they must function well enough to support to specific activity that the individual is performing more over different activity make different demands upon the organism with respect to circulatory, respiratory, metabolic and neurologic process which are specific to the activity.

High level of performance in sports and games might be dependent upon the physiological make up and it was recognized that physiological proficiency was needed for the high level performance. How much athletic ability present in a particular person is attributable to genetics, and how much is determined by training and other adaptations made by the athlete.

Physiological system is highly adaptable to exercise. Each task has major physiological components and fitness for the task require effective functioning of the appropriate system. Involvement in systematic programme of training brings about desirable changes in physiological ability which enhances the athlete's performance in his sports.

Most of the researchers, coaches and teachers of physical education emphasize that a player or an athlete must possess such characteristics of the body which suit him/her the most in his/her sport. The physiological characteristics are acknowledged to be

6

fundamental and significant for an Individual's development to achieve Olympic level performance in any sports discipline.

The use of scientific methods and techniques in the search and selection of potential athletes is a matter of routine in most of the developed countries. Especially in India unfortunately, selection process lacks proper attention and gravity, consequently, the sportsmen are selected from available pool, mainly in the basis of their previous performance in sports competitions. It is not recognized whether the available "talent" has a scope for further improvement. The coaches and experts have a call for fresh look at the methods for the selection of players. In the Indian context, therefore, it is necessary to modify selection procedure to identify talent at the right time or as early as possible. The body structure of a sportsman has tremendous influence on his physiological performance. This fact calls upon the coaches, trainers and physical education teachers to give due consideration to various physiological components of a sports men while selecting them for participating in competition. For superior performance in any sports competition an athlete may, therefore, be selected on the basis of the body size. But coaches must remain in touch with the proven and established methods of training to get a better performance from sportsmen.

Blood Pressure

Blood pressure, measured with a blood pressure cuff and stethoscope by a nurse or other healthcare provider, is the force of the blood pushing against the artery walls.

Each time the heart beats, it pumps blood into the arteries, resulting in the highest blood pressure, the systolic pressure, as the heart contracts, and the lowest blood pressure, the diastolic pressure, as the heart relaxes.

Most people think of high blood pressure, also known as hypertension, as a condition that affects older people. This may have been true in the past, but these days, high blood pressure affects people of all ages including young children.

Why is high blood pressure in children a growing problem? What can you do to protect your child from this threat? The first step is to learn all one can about high blood pressure in children, its causes, consequences, and treatment.

Resting Heart Rate

Athletes use their resting heart rate as a baseline fitness gauge. It occurs when a person is in a relaxed state, such as right after getting out of bed. The resting heart rate for an average male ranges from 60 to 80 beats per minute. It is slightly higher for women, 70 to 90 beats per minute. Well-conditioned athletes might have resting heart rates into the 40s.

High-level hockey players fall into a similar range and even recreational players have lower resting heart rates normal for people in their age group. A Canadian study on the cardiovascular condition of recreational hockey players noted that the average resting heart rate for its study group was 59.

BMI

Hockey players typically have more muscle mass than other athletes in high cardio sports. The typical BMI index for obesity would not apply.

Other sports such as track & field's Shot Put, Discus or Javelin would also have a higher BMI number due to the muscle necessary to hurl objects of varying weight a great distance. Most Olympic gold medal winners in these events have high BMI numbers yet low body fat ratios. Hockey is unique in that all players must have both foot speed and muscle mass to be effective. The higher muscle mass distorts the BMI index for Hockey players by an estimated 8 - 12%.

Peak Flow Rate

A "normal" peak flow rate is based on a person's age, height, sex and race. A standardized "normal" may be obtained from a chart comparing the patient with a population without breathing problems.

A patient can figure out what is normal for them, based on their own peak flow rate. Therefore, it is important for you and your healthcare provider to discuss what is considered "normal" for you

Peak flow meter is a portable, inexpensive, hand-held device used to measure how air flows from your lungs in one "fast blast." In other words, the meter measures your ability to push air out of your lungs.

Peak flow meters may be provided in two ranges to measure the air pushed out of your lungs. A low range peak flow meter is for small children, and a standard range peak flow meter is for older children, teenagers and adults. An adult has much larger airways than a child and needs the larger range.

Aerobic Capacity

A game of hockey involves aerobic power, as the game lasts for 70 minutes, short bursts of running (speed) followed by rapid recovery periods of lower intensity.

A game of hockey demands that players have an adequate aerobic power capacity to be able to play continuously for the duration of the game. Reilly and Borrie, (1992) analysed the physiological cost of energy expenditure of playing hockey and placed it in the category of 'heavy exercise' with reported oxygen consumption (VO_2) values during a game of 2.26 Lrnin. Boy1e et al (1994) studied the competitive demands of elite male field hockey using heart rate and VO_{2max}. They found that the mean O_2 uptake during competition was 48.2 ± 5.2 ml/kg/min which is commensurate with 78% of the group's mean maximal oxygen uptake of 61.8 ± 1.8 ml/kg/min.

These studies reflect that hockey places a heavy demand on the aerobic system and requires players to expend energy at relatively high levels. Fatigue, exhaustion or lack of stamina is limiting factors in a game of hockey and it could be classified as an endurance sport similar to soccer (Berg et al, 1985). This requires the aerobic power systems in the body to be conditioned to deliver the energy requirements.

Garry et al. after an intensive study of anthropometric measurements of Olympic athletes concluded that top level performance in particular events demands particular size of the body and shape, other aspects being similar. They established strong relationship between the structure of an athlete and specific task (event in which he excelled). Clear physical proto type exists for optimal performance at Olympic level.

Anthropometry

Physique and anthropometric variables play an important role in field hockey. Since lots of movements and skills are involved in playing field hockey therefore, a high level of physical demand is required for match play. As the players have to cover a big area in the ground during attack and defence therefore, the game demands for aerobic fitness. A high number of accelerations and decelerations, associated with the large number of changes in direction of play create an additional load to the muscles involved as in field hockey, those players better suited to cope with the demands of the game reach the elite level. Moreover, power and strength has great impact over the game, which is required during sprinting and in execution of various skills with the ball.

Anthropometry is the measurement of man and consists primarily in the measurement of the dimensions of the body. Anthropometry has also been defined as the science of measurement applied to the human body and includes measurements of height, weight, and selected body and limb girths. The use of anthropometry is a standardized method to compare bodybuilders and other athletes in the areas of muscle, body proportionality, and fat tissue. A first area of assessment is body composition. Bodybuilding, unlike performance sports, is characterized by aesthetics and by body dimensions.

Anthropometrical and physiological variables play a dominant role especially at higher level of sports competitions. The scholar is of opinion that arm length, leg length, thigh girth, body fat percentage, body mass index, peak flow rate, blood pressure, and aerobic capacity may be basic pre- requisites for attaining top-level performance in Hockey.

Anthropometric measurements are dimensions of the structure of the human body taken at specific sites to give measures of girth and width. They include the body size and body proportions. Measurements of body size include such descriptive information's as height, weight, and surface area. When the measures of body proportions describe relationship between height, weight, among lengths, widths and girths of various body segments it has been observed that top athletes in some sports tend to have those proportions that biologically aid the performance. Human performance is a composition of many variables such as structure of the body, the specific measurements of the limbs, circumferences, breadth and body build. Since motor performance is an outcome of various variables, there may be a direct relationship between certain specific measurements and motor performance. The type of individual's structure is an essential factor in his motor performance. Evidence of this is quite common observe the well proportionate physique of boxers and gymnasts, the super structure of great basketball players, the muscularity of top class football players, the wiriness of champion distance runners and the massive built of shot put and discus throwers. Therefore, anthropometric measurements of an individual player play a dominant role in high level sports performance.

There are a number of international studies investigating the physiological characteristics of elite hockey players (Bhanot and Sidhu, 1981; Sidhu, et ai, 1984; Reily and Seaton, 1990; Cibich, 1991; Reilly and Borrie, 1992; Shegril, Singh and Tung, 1992; Boyle, et ai, 1994). There is only one study that has described the anthropometric and physiological characteristics of elite male hockey players in South Africa (Scott, 1991). The findings in these studies confirm that field hockey requires a Wide variety of physical attributes for successful performance. Anthropometric and physiological characteristics have been shown to vary with field positions in senior hockey, (Withers et al, 1977; Kansal, Verna, Sidhu

11

and Sohal, 1983; Sidhu *et al,* 1984; Scott, 1991). A further aim of the current study is to determine if anthropometric and physiological characteristics differ according to field position in junior hockey.

The physical activity and athletic training can also change body composition. The economy of work performance depends on ratio of these components. The changes in body composition during increasing age depend partly on one's genetic development and partly no functional aerobic capacity. The aerobic working capacity is relatively higher at younger ages, which decrease with decreasing lean body mass, with increasing age.

The body composition studies have been conducted very extensively on the athletes. The examination of body fat and skin-folds at selected sites is most important in them. It has been found that the athletes who were lean or less fatty but heavy because of a well-developed musculature were superior in performance in certain competitive sports. On the other hand he athletes who had substantial amount of adipose tissue have permanently increased energy demands owing to the inert weight of fat, thus making the work more difficult to perform in such activities where the body has to be projected as in jumping movements, or propelled against activity over long distance and in distance running.

Height

Height is an important factor in many sports. In volleyball and basketball height is an advantage whereas in hockey it may be somewhat of a disadvantage to be tall because of the stooping posture (Scott, 1991). In male hockey players, the mean height in the Indian winning team at the Tokyo Olympics was 1.73m (Hirata, 1966). The Pakistani and non-Asian teams were taller. The small size of Indian international players reported in other studies reflects the smaller stature of the Asian population rather than elite hockey players (Bhanot & Sidhu, 1981). The elite South African players had a mean height of 1.76m (Scott, 1991). The mean height of female hockey players tends to range from 1.62 to 1.65m

Arm Length

Scott (1991) felt that because hockey involves playing with a hockey stick to control and pass the ball, arm length would be a factor affecting performance. However, in her study there appeared to be no relationship between arm length and playing ability and therefore arm length was not included in the current study.

Body Weight

Body mass is also an important factor in hockey, as there are positional differences in body mass between forwards, backs and goalkeepers (Sidhu et al, 1984). Amongst top level Indian women hockey players, Kansal et al, (1980) found that goalkeepers and backs were heaviest followed by halves and forwards respectively. Malhorta, Joseph and Gupta, (1974) found that the goalkeepers were shortest, had the lowest percent lean bodyweight and the highest percent body fat; the forwards were the lightest, with the least percent body fat and the highest lean body weight, the backs were the tallest with percentage body fats and lean body mass intermediate between goalkeepers and forwards.

Percentage Of Body Fat

Scott (1991), in her study on elite male hockey players, found that they had a fairly low percentage body fat of 11.1%, whereas, Withers *et al* (1977) found that South Australian state male hockey players had a percentage body fat of 16.7%. Elite female hockey players had a percentage body fat ranging from 15.7-18.9% in the Canadian.

Olympic Hockey team (Ready and Vander Merwe, 1986) Withers and Roberts (1981) reported a value of 25.3%, Reilly *et al* (1985), reported a figure of 25.8% for Welsh national players whilst values of 23 and 22.9% were found in English elite squad and country players, respectively (Reilly and Bretherton, 1986). Withers *et al (1987)*, found a mean of 20.2% for South Australian players. Reilly and Secher (1990) reported a spread of mean values in the literature for female hockey players ranging from 16 to 26%. The lower values were found in the elite players close to peak fitness for international

13

tournaments. In summary it would appear that a lower level of body fat is not essential for elite performance. However, it must be noted that the accurate measurement of skinfolds, using a skinfold calliper is dependent on the operators that are taking the measurements and therefore, an inter-operator variability of measurements will be expected. Therefore, any comparison between studies need to viewed with caution.

An interesting area on futurism or futuristic which makes an attempt of scientifically examine the future has attracted us all. In the field of sports also sports scientist have been making the effort of prediction the success of sportsperson during competition. The prediction is usually based on a scientific study of physiological and anthropometrical factor of the sports person.

The variables that contribute to the successful performance in any sports event are broadly classified as physiological and anthropometrical. Physiological variable resting heart rate, peak flow rate, blood pressure (Systolic and Diastolic), Body Mass Index (BMI), Aerobic Capacity etc some of the anthropometric variable height, weight, arm length, leg length, thigh girth, body fat percentage etc.

Anthropometric measurement may be classified as-

1. Linear measurement such as height, weight, arm length, leg length etc.
2. Circumference such as thigh girth etc.
3. Skin fold such as triceps, biceps, subscapula, suprailliac, etc.

Physiological variables may be defined as those variables which are directly linked with various physiological systems such as resting heart rate, blood pressure, peak flow rate, fat percentage, aerobic capacity.

Physiological variable such as aerobic capacity, peak flow rate, blood pressure, body mass index, resting heart rate and other should be given due to weightage of the selection of the hockey player. Aerobic capacity was consider as one of the important variable for efficient performance in hockey game as hockey player has to make nonstop continuous movement during competition. Aerobic capacity enable a person to make for a prolonged period of the time without undue fatigue with the help of oxygen which is collected, transported and utilised by lungs, blood and muscles respectively physical activity of any nature is directly related to energy supplying system which in turn is the aerobic capacity of an individual. High level of hockey performance not only depend on physical fitness like speed, flexbility, strength , power, agility, endurance but also physiological and anthropometrical variable in addition to technique and tactics of a player or a team.

Sports performance is the sum of numerous factors which can vary from individual to individual, even if ultimately they achieve similar results in competition. Deficient person can be compensated for being superior technique, inadequate sprinting speed by superior endurance or inferior technique by aggressiveness. A few centimetres and fraction of seconds decide between record performances, victory or defeat in tough international competitions; for this reason it is very important to identify and fully realize each individuals potential.

Whether there can be an end to human efficiency relating to his performance in sports, it is really a extremely difficult question to answer because, records are being shattered every day. To the casual observer, it would seem that we must indeed reach the point where further improvement in performance is almost impossible. But this is not to be for the existing trends clearly show that improvement is without doubt, possible. May be that the more precise ways of measuring performance are used. Knowledge obtained from progress of past records over the year should permit one to speculate on the future changes likely to occur.

It has become a necessity to identify and select a future elite athlete right in childhood cr adolescence. It makes many years of intensive regular training till an international sports performance level is achieved. The children, who are selected for elite sports activities require suitable conditions and sports facilities equipment of high quality, a rational style of life and the service of experts including a sports physician, a well educated and experienced coach etc. Such conditions can be created for selected children only. Therefore, the correct identification, selection and placement of young talent is becoming important everywhere.

On the basis of above mentioned facts, it was considered worthwhile to investigate the relationship of selected Physiological and Anthropometric variables for prediction of Hockey Performance. Moreover, the present study would high light some of the important Physiological and Anthropometric variables determinants which may have to bear in mind while looking for the selection of talented Field Hockey and also to develop these components through the systematic training programme.

Physiological and anthropometric variable help the performer for better performance.

Statement of the Problem

The title of the study hereby stated as "Predicting excellence in junior and sub junior elite field hockey players on the basis of selected anthropometric and physiological variables".

Objectives of the Study

1. The objective of the study was to characterize the anthropometric and physiological variables of Junior and Sub junior Field hockey players.

2. The objective of the study was to find out correlation between dependent variable (Hockey performance) and independent variables (selected anthropometric and physiological variables).

3. Another objective of the study was to find out joint contribution of independent variables (selected anthropometric and physiological variables) in predicting dependent variable (Hockey performance).

4. To establish regression equation for predicting dependent variable (Hockey performance) on the basis of independent variables (selected anthropometric and physiological variables).

Delimitations

1. The study was delimited to male field hockey players.
2. The study was delimited to 30 Junior and 30 Sub-Junior field hockey players.
3. The study was further delimited to the following selected Anthropometric and Physiological variables-:

- **Anthropometric Variables**
    1. Standing Height
    2. Weight
    3. Arm Length
    4. Leg Length
    5. Thigh Girth
    6. Body Fat Percentage

- **Physiological Variables**
    1. Blood pressure
        a. Systolic Blood Pressure
        b. Diastolic Blood Pressure
    2. Peak Flow Rate
    3. Resting Heart Rate
    4. Aerobic Capacity
    5. Body Mass Index (BMI)

4. The study was delimited to different levels of participation of field hockey players i.e.-
    I. National Camp
    II. National

Limitations

1. Personal habits of the subjects and their state of mind as well as emotional state, stress and other factors which may have effect on the result of this study and could not be controlled, it was considered as one of the limitation of the present study.

2. Certain factors like diet, daily routine habits, facilities, training, climatic conditions etc may effect on the results of the study was also considered as the limitation of the study.

Hypothesis

Based on the evidence available in the literature and on the basis of discussion with experts, the following hypothesis were formulated-

1. There shall not be any significant relationship between dependent variable (Hockey performance) and independent variables (anthropometric and physiological variables).

2. There shall not be any significant joint contribution of independent variables (selected anthropometric and physiological variables) in relation to dependent variable (Hockey performance).

Definitions and Explanation of Terms

Prediction

It is the statement of claim that a particular event will be occurring in the future.

Anthropometry

The study of human body measurement for use in anthropological classification and comparison.

Elite Player

In the present study, the term elite player is used for the players who were shortlisted from four semi-finalist teams.

Standing Height

Human height is the distance from the bottom of the feet to the top of the head in a human body standing erect.

Weight

Body weight is the measurement of physical as material frame of the material organism (women/men) as determined by means of weighing.

Arm Length

Linear distance between the acromion to tip of the third finger.

Leg Length

From the end of the spinal column to the floor also taken from greater trochanter to floor.

Thigh Girth

An anthropometric measurement that is the circumference of the thigh (usually the right) 1-2 cm below the protuberance of the gluteal muscles on the thigh. The measurement is taken when the subject is standing erect with feet slightly apart and with weight equally distributed on both feet.

Blood Pressure

Blood pressure (BP) is the pressure exerted by circulating blood upon the walls of blood vessels, and is one of the principal vital signs. When used without further specification, "blood pressure" usually refers to the arterial pressure of the systemic circulation. During each heartbeat, blood pressure varies between a maximum (systolic) and a minimum (diastolic) pressure.

Peak Flow Rate

Rate of the flow of air per minute at the peak expiratory condition.

Resting Heart Rate

Heart rate is the number of heartbeats per unit of time, typically expressed as beats per minute (BPM). Heart rate can vary as the body's need to absorb oxygen and excrete carbon dioxide changes, such as during exercise or sleep.

Aerobic Capacity

Aerobic capacity describes the functional capacity of the cardio- respiratory system, (the heart, lungs and blood vessels). Aerobic capacity is defined as the maximum amount of oxygen the body can use during a specified period, usually during intense exercise.

Body Mass Index (BMI)

Body mass index is a method of estimating a person body fat percentage based upon simple weight and height.

$$BMI = Weight\ (kg)\ /\ Height\ (m)^2$$

Body Fat Percentage

Fat percentage is the percentage of lean body mass subtracted from total body weight.

Significance of the Study

The present study may be helpful in the following manner:-

1. The study may reveal true facts about Indian junior and sub-junior hockey players.

2. The study may help the physical education teachers and coaches to scan the prospective male Indian hockey players of different levels.

3. It will be helpful to differentiate anthropometric and physiological variables possessed by different levels of junior and sub-junior hockey players.

4. The study would make some positive addition to increase the knowledge connected with the performance of the hockey players at different level of competition. The result of study may highlight the selected anthropometric and physiological variables of hockey players.

5. The study may provide guide lines for the coaches to develop a specific talent identification programs for young hockey players.

6. The study will develop a criterion for objective measurement of the hockey players based on anthropometric and physiological variables.

7. Results may be helpful for self-assessment of the junior and sub-junior hockey players.

8. The study may reveal the role-played by some crucial factors which determine success of hockey player.

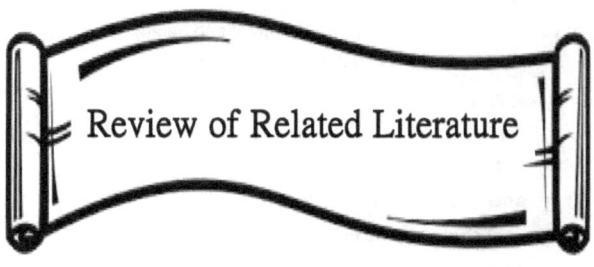

Chapter - 2

Review of Related Literature

In this chapter a serious and scholarly attempt has been made by the research scholar to go through the literature related to the study. The relevant studies of specific importance are cited below.

Dravin, Singh Y, Bangari D (2013) conducted study to compare selected physical fitness components, skill level and anthropometric measurements among selected hockey players. For the study, total forty male hockey players were selected from following places of Uttar Pradesh i.e. Lucknow, Varanasi, Saifai and Shajahanpur. Ten players from each city were selected through purposive sampling technique. The anthropometric measurements were taken on each subject using standard methodology given by Weiner and Laurie (1969) which were Height (cm), Weight (kg) and Body Mass Index. The selected Physical fitness test items used for the study were- pull ups and shuttle run and for measuring skill level, SAI hockey skill test was used. The only selected item from the hockey skill test was shooting the target. Analysis of Variance was used to find out the significant difference in selected physical fitness, anthropometric and skill test variables among the players. The results in relation to anthropometric measurements i.e. height, weight and BMI were found almost similar in all players of different selected places. Statistically, result was found insignificant but Varanasi hockey players were found taller as compared to other

21

selected places. Significant differences were found in selected Physical fitness i.e. arm and shoulder strength and speed. Post hoc test indicated Shajahanpur players were better in arm and shoulder strength as compared to Varanasi and Lucknow hockey players. In level of selected hockey skill i.e. ball shooting ability, no significant difference was found among all.

Sidhu J.S.(2013) conducted study to find out relationship of selected anthropometric variables of upper limbs to the performance in male hockey players for the purpose of the study 35 player were selected who had participated at Punjab agricultural university in 2009. Their age ranged from 17 to 25 years. Anthropometric variable were measured by anthropometric kit and performance was measured by rating from expert/judges. Data were collected for weight, height, sitting height, arm length, shoulder diameter, elbow diameter, chest circumferences, upper arm circumferences, body fat percentage with the help of anthropometric kit. To find out relationship of selected anthropometric variables of upper limbs to the performance in male hockey players multiple correlations was applied. The analysis of data revealed positive and significant relationship between selected anthropometric variables of upper limbs (weight, height, sitting height, arm length, shoulder diameter, elbow diameter, chest circumferences, upper arm circumferences,) to the performance in male hockey players. The negative and insignificant relationship found between skin fold measurement (triceps, sub-scapula, suprailliac) to the performance in male hockey players.

Tarverdizadeh, B., Azarbayjani, M.A. (2012) conducted a study to determine the relationships between selected anthropometric with physical and motor fitness measures in elite Iranian soccer players. Among the players of national team, 60 elite men were selected voluntary as an overall sample. The anthropometric measures included, body mass index (BMI), fat %, weight, lean body mass, height and also chest, leg and thigh circumferences and body composition from total of 60 elite players. Also measurements (sectioned as: skin folds, girths, lengths, and

22

breadths) were made for each player. The procedure involved three measures at each site to calculate a mean value and used to relate with fitness variables. The physical and motor fitness tests used were: ergo jump, vertical jump, agility, flexibility, speed and reaction time. Mean calculated scores for all players were obtained. Regression analyses indicated significant correlation between certain variables of Fitness tests and variables of anthropometric estimation statistics. Knowing these relationships provides us with valuable predictive information about player's Capabilities in sport. Results showed between have less body mass index (BMI), less fat%, greater lean body mass , great leg and thigh circumferences were significantly related to better speed, agility, ergo jump and vertical jump . Also observed greater height with vertical jump ($p < 0.05$) and relationships between agility and flexibility to less fat observed too. Regression analysis for all variables demonstrated a significant relationship between some parameters. These findings suggest that we can predict some variables of anthropometric or physical and motor fitness by other parameters.

Francise. Holway, Marianoseara (2011) conducted a study (a) to establish the anthropometric characteristics of elite junior Argentine male field hockey players; (b) to look for differences in physique, years of playing and birth-date effect between the final players selected to make up the team and those who were not selected out of the original pre-selected sample; and(c) to establish whether there are any differences in proportional limb lengths between elite junior hockey players and a local reference sample. Thirty five elite Argentine junior field hockey players pre-selected to form the base of the national junior team for the 2005 Junior World Cup (Age19.0±1.0 years; weight 70.7±5.4 kg; height176.4±6.4 cm). A full anthropometric battery including lengths, heights, breadths, girths, and skinfolds, plus number of years playing and date of birth was recorded. No statistically significant differences were found in skeletal structural dimensions when compared to a reference sample, nor between finally selected and non-selected players in anthropometric dimensions, playing history ($P = .11$) and relative-

23

age effect (P = .11). Conclusion: Male field hockey is a sport with normal bone-structural requirements, and with a lack of birth-date effect in Argentina.

Karkare A., (2011) conducted study to compare anthropometric measurements and body composition of hockey players with respect to their playing position. Two hundred and ten junior national hockey players seventy each from half line, back line and forward line was selected different state of india. Anthropometric measurements including height, weight, diameter, breadth, girth, and skinfold thickness was taken from entire subjects. Body composition was measured with the help of Matiegka's method (1921).To find out significant difference statistical method one way ANOVA was performed. Results found that, hockey players playing in different position found to differ on some anthropometric measurements and body composition.

Lythe J, Kilding A.E (2011) conducted study to determine the physical demands of elite men's field hockey using modern time-motion analysis techniques. 18 elite male players (age: 24.4 ± 4.5 yrs) participated in 5 matches, during which physical outputs of players were quantified using GPS units and heart rate monitors. The mean total distance covered by each individual player was 6798 ± 2009 m. Mean total distance covered per position for 70 min (position (70)) was 8160 ± 428 m. Distance covered per position (70) decreased by 4.8% between the 1 (st)and 2 (nd) halves (P < 0.05). Fullbacks covered significantly less total distance than all other positions (P < 0.05). High-intensity running (>19 km.h (-1)) comprised 6.1% (479 ± 108 m) of the total distance covered and involved 34 ± 12 sprints per player, with an average duration of 3.3 s. Average HR was higher in the 1 (st) half (86.7% HR (max)) than the 2 (nd) half, (84.4% HR (max)), though this was not significant (P = 0.06). The results suggest that modern day elite field hockey is a physically demanding team sport. Quantification of the demands and outputs of players at this level provides a useful framework on which to develop conditioning practices. The difference in physical outputs observed for some positions suggests position-specific conditioning is required at the elite level.

Manna I, Khanna G. L, Dhara P. C., *(2010)* conducted study to find out the effect of a pre competition training on selected physiological and health-related variables of Indian field hockey players of different age groups. 120 field hockey players volunteered for the study. Players were divided equally (n=30) into four groups: (i) under 16 years (U16), (ii) under 19 years (U19), (iii) under 23 years (U23), (iv) senior (SR). The training sessions consisted of three phases: a) Transition Phase (TP, 4 weeks), b) Preparatory Phase (PP, 8 weeks), and c) Competitive Phase (CP, 4 weeks) and completed 4hrs/day; 5 days/week. A significantly higher ($P<0.05$) lean body mass (LBM), VO_{2max}, anaerobic power (AP), strength, urea, uric acid, HDL-C; and a lower ($P<0.05$) body fat, hemoglobin (Hb), total cholesterol (TC), triglyceride (TG) and LDL-C were observed in some groups in PP and CP when compared to that of TP. When comparing different age groups, significantly ($P<0.05$) higher LBN, AP, strength, Hb, TC, TG, HDL-C and LDL-C; and lower ($P<0.05$) body fat and VO_{2max} were noted in U23 and senior players than the U16 and U19 players. This study would provide useful information for training and selection of field hockey players of different age groups.

Manna I, Khanna G. L, Dhara P. C., **(2010)** conducted study to investigate the effect of training on selected anthropometric, physiological and biochemical variables of elite field hockey players. A total of 30 Indian male field hockey players (age: 23.00-30.00 yrs) volunteered for this study. The training sessions were divided into 2 phases (a) Preparatory Phase (PP, 8 weeks) and (b) Competitive Phase (CP, 4 weeks). The training programme consisted of aerobic, anaerobic and skill development, and were completed 4 hrs/day; 5 days/week. Selected variables were measured at zero level (baseline data, BD) and at the end of PP and CP. A significant increase ($P<0.05$) in LBM, back and hand grip strength, serum level of urea, uric acid and HDLC; and a significant decrease ($P<0.05$) in body fat, sub-maximal exercise heart rate and recovery heart rate, hemoglobin, total cholesterol, triglyceride and LDLC were noted in PP and CP of

25

training when compare to BD. No significant change was noted in stature, body mass, HRmax, resting heart rate, VO2max and anaerobic power of the players after the training. Since the data on field hockey players are limited in India, the present study may provide useful information to the coaches to develop their training programme.

Singh M, Singh M. K, Singh K., (2010) conducted study to determine the anthropometric measurements and body composition of field hockey teams of India, Pakistan and Sri Lanka. A total of 53 field hockey players from three teams were studied. The participants' height was measured using the standard anthropometric rod, while their weight was measured with a portable weighing machine. Widths and diameters of body parts were measured using digital caliper. Girths and lengths were taken with a steel tape. Grip strength was measured with a hand dynamometer. Skin fold thickness measurements were taken using the Harpenden caliper at 4 sites (biceps, triceps, subscapular and suprailliac). The percentage of fat was calculated from the sum of 4 measurements of skin fold thickness. It was found that there were no significant differences in height and weight among the three teams, with the Pakistani players recording a slightly higher weight. The Pakistan team had a significantly higher upper arm length (p<0.05) and bi-hummers diameter (p<0.05) as compared to the India and the Sri Lanka teams. The Sri Lanka team had significantly less wrist circumference (p<0.05), hand width (p<0.05) and lean body mass (p<0.05) as compared to the India and the Pakistan teams. The India team had significantly less % body fat (p<0.05) than the other two teams. More data would be of interest to document the changes in anthropometry and body composition during the season and out of season and also to attempt an analysis of characteristics specific to field positions

Chauhan et al. (2009) conducted study to develop the regression equation for the prediction of sprinting ability of secondary school boys. The data was collected from the boys of age range between 16 to 18 years(X=17) by anthrop meter, skin fold calliper, venire calliper and steel tape. The Pearson product movement method for correlations, Wherry Do Little method for calculation multiple correlation and development of regression equation were utilized. Linear measurements, i.e., height, leg length, fore leg length, total arm length, thigh length and foot length, girth measurements i.e., shoulder, chest, abdomen, hip, thigh and calf, body diameters i.e. biacromial, bicirstal and ankle diameters, subscapular and thigh skinfolds, fat weight and lean body mass, body weight and age has significant and negative correlations with sprinting ability. The multiple correlation of a selected combination of variables i.e. length, biacromial diameter and lean body mass with sprinting ability have been found highly significant. The developed multiple correlations are of sufficient size and the regression equation can be put in the prediction of sprinting ability of secondary school boys.

Quinney HA, Dewart R, Game A, Snydmiller G, Warburton D, Bell G (2008) conducted study to investigate the physiological profile of a National Hockey League (NHL) team over a period of 26 years. All measurements were made at a similar time of year (pre-season) in 703 male (mean age +/- SD = 24 +/- 4 y) hockey players. The data were analyzed across years, between positions (defensemen, forwards, and goaltenders), and between what were deemed successful and non-successful years using a combination of points acquired during the season and play-off success. Most anthropometric (height, mass, and BMI) and physiological parameters (absolute and relative VO_2 peak, relative peak 5 s power output, abdominal endurance, and combined grip strength) showed a gradual increase over the 26 year period. Defensemen were taller and heavier, had higher absolute VO_2 peak, and had greater combined grip strength than forwards and goaltenders. Forwards were younger and had higher values for relative VO_2 peak. Goaltenders were shorter, had less body mass, a higher sum of skinfolds, lower VO_2 peak, and better flexibility. The overall pre-season fitness profile was not related to team success. In conclusion, this study revealed that the fitness profile for a professional NHL ice-

27

hockey team exhibited increases in player size and anaerobic and aerobic fitness parameters over a 26 year period that differed by position. However, this evolution of physiological profile did not necessarily translate into team success in this particular NHL franchise.

Gravina, et al. (2008) conducted a study to identify differences in the anthropometric and physiological characteristics of first team and reserve young soccer players (10-14 years old) at both the beginning and end of the soccer season. Body composition was calculated by measuring weight, height, skinfold, limb circumference and joint diameter. Vo2max was estimated by Astrand's test. Sprint and jump tests were also performed. In general, first team players (FTPs) were taller and leaner. However, the most relevant difference that we found at the beginning of the season was that FTPs had shorter sprint times than reserves in the 30-m test (both flat and with 10 cones). Moreover, these differences in sprint time were more marked at the end of the season. In addition, jump test performance by the reserves declined from the beginning to the end of the season. These results indicate that sprint time is an important factor associated with selection as an FTP between the ages of 10 and 14 years. The progression of the FTPs during the course of the season is better than that of the reserves and is associated with a different degree of growth and maturity. These findings should be taken into account by trainers and coaches to avoid a bias against late maturing or younger soccer players.

Elferink, Visscher, et al (2007) conducted study to reveal performance characteristics, which may have power for predicting future elite field hockey players, we made a comparison between 30 elite and 35 sub-elite youth players in terms of anthropometric, physiological, technical, tactical and psychological characteristics measured on three occasions, each separated by a time interval of one year. Mean age of the players on the first measurement was 14.2 years (sd = 1.1). Repeated measures analyses of covariance with factors of performance level and measurement, and with age as a covariate, showed that the elite players scored better than the sub-elite players on technical and tactical variables. Female elite youth players also scored better on interval endurance capacity, motivation and confidence. Future elite players seem to excel in tactical skills by the age of 14 already. They also stand out in specific technical skills and develop these together with the interval endurance capacity better than sub-elite youth players in the two subsequent years. It will be interesting to follow these players until they reach elite status in adulthood to verify these conclusions.

Gil, S.M. et al. (2007) conducted this study to establish the anthropometric and physiological profiles of young non elite soccer players according to their playing position, and to determine their relevance for the selection process. Two hundred forty-one male soccer players who were members of the Getxo Arenas Club (Bizkaia) participated in this study. Players, age 17.31 (± 2.64) years, range 14-21 years, were classified into the following groups: forwards (n = 56), midfielders (n = 79), defenders (n = 77), and goalkeepers (n = 29). Anthropometric variables of participants (height, weight, body mass index, 6 skinfolds, 4 diameters, and 3 perimeters) were measured. Also, their somatotype and body composition (weights and percentages of fat, bone, and muscle) were calculated. Participants performed the Astrand test to estimate their absolute and relative O2max, an endurance test, sprint tests (30 meters flat and 30 meters with 10 cones) and 3 jump tests (squat jump, counter movement jump and drop jump). Forwards were the leanest, presenting the highest percentage of muscle. They were the best performers in all the physiological tests, including endurance, velocity, agility, and power. In contrast, goalkeepers were found to be the tallest and the heaviest players. They also had the largest fat skinfolds and the highest fat percentage, but their aerobic capacity was the lowest. In the selection process, agility and the jump tests were the most discriminating for forwards. In contrast, agility, height, and endurance were the key factors for midfielders. The defenders group was characterized by a lower quantity of fat. Thus, we may conclude that anthropometric and physiological differences exist among soccer players who play in different positions. These differences fit with their different workload in a game. Therefore, training programs should include specific sessions for each positional role.

Chauhan, (2006) conducted study to determine the relationship between anthropometric variables and the middle distance running performance and also to develop regression equation for the prediction of performance of the athletes between the age range of 18 and 30 years. The data was collected from 1500 meters middle distance runners as subjects of the study by using anthropometer, skinfold caliper, vernier calliper and steel tape. The product movement method for correlation and wherry do little method for calculating multiple correlation and development of regression equation were utilized. Linear measurements, i.e., height, leg length, thigh length, total arm length, girth measurements, i.e., biacromial and ankle diameter, thigh(negative) and calf skinfold, lean body mass and age have positive and significant correlations with middle distance running performance. The multiple correlation of selected combination of variables (i.e. height, thigh girth, biacromial diameter and thigh skinfold) with middle distance running performance have been found significant but the multiple correlation is not of sufficient size, (so the regression equation developed cannot be put in the prediction of middle distance running performance).

Duncan, et al. (2006) conducted study to investigate the anthropometric and physiological characteristics of junior elite volleyball players. Twenty five national level volleyball players (mean (SD) age 17.5 (0.5) years) were assessed on a number of physiological and anthropometric variables. Somatotype was assessed using the Health-Carter method, body composition (% body fat, % muscle mass) was assessed using surface anthropometry, leg strength was assessed using a leg and back dynamometer, low back and hamstring flexibility was assessed using the sit and reach test and the vertical jump was used as a measure of lower body power. Maximal oxygen uptake was predicted using the 20 m multistage fitness test. Setters were more ectomorphic (p<0.05) and less mesomorphic (p<0.01) than centres. Mean (SD) of somatotype (endomorphy, mesomorphy, ectomorphy) for setters and centres was 2.6 (0.9), 1.9 (1.1), 5.3 (1.2) and 2.2 (0.8), 3.9 (1.1), 3.6 (0.7) respectively. Hitters had significantly greater low back and hamstring flexibility than opposites. Mean (SD) for sit and reach was 19.3 (8.3) cm for opposites and 37 (10.7) cm for hitters. There were no other significant differences in physiological and anthropometric variables across playing positions (all p>0.05). Setters tend to be endomorphic ectomorphs, hitters and opposites tend to be balanced ectomorphs, whereas centres tend to be ectomorphic mesomorphs. These results indicated the need for sports scientists and conditioning professionals to take the body type of volleyball players into account when designing individualised position specific training programmes.

Stagno K.M, Thatcher R, Van Someren K.A., (2005) conducted study to measure the physiological profiles of elite players and observed changes throughout a season in order to provide guidelines for training. Secondly, investigate whether recent rule changes have had an impact on the physiological demands of match play. Nine English premier division male field hockey players participated in this study (mean s: age 24±4 years, body mass 80.8±5.2 kg and height 181.8±3.9 cm). Three treadmill exercise tests were performed at pre-season (T1), at the start of the competitive season (T2) and at midcompetitive season (T3), to determine the running velocity at a blood lactate concentration of 4 mmol-l^{-1} (V_{OBLA}), individual HR:VO_2 regressions, VO_{2peak}, peak running speed (PRS) and time to exhaustion. There were increases (p<0.05) between T1 and T2 in VO_{2peak} (54.0±6.3 to 60.1±7.6 ml·kg^{-1}·min^{-1}) and PRS (18.2±1.7 to 19.1±1.7 km·h^{-1}). V_{OBLA} increased from T2 to T3 (15.1±1.7 to 15.8±1.4 km·h^{-1}, p<0.05) and time to exhaustion increased from T1 to T3 (30.3±8.0 s to 33.0±5.9 s). The subjects' mean responses to competition match play were; heart rate 167±8 beats ·min^{-1}, VO_2 42.8±6.3 ml·min^{-1}·kg^{-1} and a fractional utilisation of 80±7 %. The high levels of aerobic fitness observed are consistent with the demands of the games. However, there were significant changes in fitness over the course of a training year. Recent rule changes do not seem to alter the physiological demands of match play.

Elferink-Gemser MT, Visscher C, Lemmink KA, Mulder TW (2004) conducted study to determine the relationship between multidimensional performance characteristics and level of performance in talented youth field hockey players, elite youth players (n = 38, mean age 13.2 years, s = 1.26) were compared with sub-elite youth players (n = 88, mean age 14.2 years, s = 1.26) on anthropometric, physiological, technical, tactical and psychological characteristics. Multivariate analyses with performance level and gender as factors, and age as the covariate, showed that the elite youth players scored better than the sub-elite youth players on technical (dribble performance in a peak and repeated shuttle run), tactical (general tactics; tactics for possession and non-possession of the ball) and psychological variables (motivation) (P < 0.05). The most discriminating variables were tactics for possession of the ball, motivation and performance in a slalom dribble. Age discriminated between the two groups, indicating that the elite youth players were younger than the sub-elite players. In the guidance of young talented players to the top as well as in the detection of talented players, more attention has to be paid to tactical qualities, motivation and specific technical skills.

Keogh, Justin W.L, Weber, Clare L, Dalton, Carl T.,(2003) conducted study to develop an effective testing battery for female field hockey by using anthropometric, physiological, and skill-related tests to distinguish between regional representative (Rep, n = 35) and local club level (Club, n = 39) female field hockey players. Rep players were significantly leaner and recorded faster times for the 10-m and 40-m sprints as well as the Illinois Agility Run (with and without dribbling a hockey ball). Rep players also had greater aerobic and lower body muscular power and were more accurate in the shooting accuracy test, p < 0.05. No significant differences between groups were evident for height, body mass, speed decrement in 6 x 40-m repeated sprints, handgrip strength, or pushing speed. These results incicate that %BF, sprinting speed, agility, dribbling control, aerobic and muscular power, and shooting accuracy can distinguish between female field hockey players of varying standards. Therefore talent identification programs for female field hockey should include assessments of these physical parameters.

Carolina F, Nieuwenhuis, Emanuel J. Spamer & Jaques H. A. Van R (2002) conducted study to identify kinanthropometric, motor-physical and psychological variables and specific field hockey skills that influence field hockey performance at the age of 14 to 15 years. The two top girls' field hockey teams in the North West Province (South Africa) U/15 (under 15 age group) field hockey league (n = 27), as well as the two teams who ended at the bottom of the league (n = 25), were exposed to a test battery. The 52 subjects were classified according to their league results as successful and less successful. The test battery consisted of nine field hockey skills tests, 16 kinanthropometric tests and six physical-motor ability tests and two sport psychological tests. A statistical analysis of the data was done for descriptive purposes and statistical significances between the successful and less successful players were determined. Results indicated meaningful differences in some variables. A prediction function was therefore developed consisting of eight variables that successfully distinguished between successful and less successful 14- to 15-year-old female field hockey players equation developed cannot be put in the prediction of middle distance running performance).

Wassmer D.J, Mookerjee S, (2002), conducted study to develop a descriptive profile and examine the relationships between grip strength, power and sport specific test performance in 37 elite, female collegiate field hockey players (N=8 backs, N=13 forwards, N=4 goalkeepers, N=8 midfield players, N=4 wings). The tests included circumference and limb lengths, %body fat, Margaria-Kalamen stair test, 50-yard dash test, Queen's College step test, grip strength, Illinois agility test, field hockey specific skills tests, and a coordination test. Mean (+/-SD) height, weight, percent body fat, and predicted oxygen consumption were 164.26 (+/-5.17) cm, 63.06 (+/-8.60) kg, 17.29 (+/-3.79)% and 42.87 (+/-9.08) ml x kg(-1) x min(-1), respectively. Although the goalkeepers were significantly (p<0.05) heavier and had a higher %body fat, there were no significant differences (p>0.05) between any of the player positions in height, limb length, 50-yard dash time, predicted VO(2max), grip strength, agility, or in the field hockey specific tests. There were no significant (p>0.05) correlations (r=0.03 to -0.13) between right and left grip strength and sport-specific test scores but significant (p<0.05) relationships were found between power and pushing accuracy, as well as between the 50 yard dash and coordination test, pushing power and pushing accuracy. In profiling a sample of elite collegiate field hockey players in the Unites States, the results of this study indicate that there are similarities amongst the defensive and offensive players with international level field hockey players, and that measures of power and sport specific tests are significantly correlated.

T. Reilly, J. Bangsbo and A. Franks (2000) conducted study to focus on anthropometric and physiological characteristics of soccer players with a view to establish their roles within talent detection, identification and development programmes. Top-class soccer players have to adapt to the physical demands of the game, which are multi factorial. Players may not need to have an extraordinary capacity within any of the areas of physical performance but must possess a reasonably high level within all areas. This explains why there are marked individual differences in anthropometric and physiological characteristics among top players. Various measurements have been used to evaluate specific aspects of the physical performance of both youth and adult soccer players. The positional role of a player is related to his or her physiological capacity. Thus, mid field players and full-backs have the highest maximal oxygen intakes (> 60 ml ´kg- 1 ´min- 1) and perform best in intermittent exercise tests. On the other hand, mid field players tend to have the lowest muscle strength. Although these

34

distinctions are evident in adult and elite youth players, their existence must be interpreted circumspectly in talent identification and development programmes. A range of relevant anthropometric and physiological factors can be considered which are subject to strong genetic influences (e.g. stature and maximal oxygen intake) or are largely environmentally determined and susceptible to training effects. Consequently, fitness profiling can generate a useful database against which talented groups may be compared. No single method allows for a representative assessment of a player's physical capabilities for soccer. We conclude that anthropometric and physiological criteria do have a role as part of a holistic monitoring of talented young players.

Weber C. L. and Keogh J. C. L. (2000) conducted study specific physiological and skill based characteristics may be related to the playing position of senior athletes in team sports (1-6). However, physical capacity and skill level of female junior athletes has not been related to playing position. Specialized training of forward, back and midfield hockey players at a junior representative level, may be useful for the successful transition into senior representative hockey. The present study assessed fitness and skill components of female junior and senior hockey players of the same relative standard (regional representative) and related performance values to playing position. We hypothesized that no specific performance measure is related to playing position in female junior hockey players, whereas certain components of fitness are significantly related to playing position in senior players. Physiological tests included; 10m and 40m sprint, 6 x 40m repeated sprint (7), multistage aerobic test, standing long jump, agility test, body mass, height and four skinfolds. Skill level was assessed using pushing power, dribbling and accuracy tests. Each player was ranked for athletic ability, regardless of position, by coaches and selectors. Results indicated that differences exist between senior and junior female hockey players in several performance measures. No obvious relationship between playing position and any performance measure was demonstrated in junior hockey players. In contrast, senior hockey players demonstrated that certain characteristics of physical ability are related to playing position. We conclude that playing position is related to particular physiological based characteristics in senior players only.

Gabbett (2000) conducted study to investigate the physiological and anthropometric characteristics of amateur rugby league players. Thirty five amateur rugby league players (19 forwards and 16 backs) were measured for height, body mass, percentage body fat (sum of four skinfolds), muscular power (vertical jump), speed (10 m and 40 m sprint) and maximal aerobic power (multistage fitness test). Data were also collected on match frequency, training status, playing experience and employment related physical activity levels. The 10 m and 40 m sprint, vertical jump, percentage body fat and multistage fitness test results were 20-42% poorer than previously reported for professional rugby league players. Compared with forwards, backs had significantly (p<0.01) lower body mass (79.7 (74.7-84.7) kg v 90.8 (86.2-95.4) kg) and significantly (p<0.01) greater speed during the 40 m sprint (6.45 (6.35-6.55) v 6.79 (6.69-6.89) seconds). Values for percentage body fat, vertical jump, 10 m sprint and maximal aerobic power were not significantly different (p>0.05) between forwards and backs. When compared with professional rugby league players, the training status of amateur rugby league players was 30-53% lower with players devoting less than three hours a week to team training sessions and about 30 minutes a week to individual training sessions. The training time devoted to the development of muscular power (about 13 minutes a week), speed (about eight minutes a week), and aerobic fitness (about 34 minutes a week) did not differ significantly (p>0.05) between forwards and backs. At the time of the field testing, players had participated, on average, in a 60 minute match every eight days. The physiological and anthropometric characteristics of amateur rugby league players are poorly developed. These findings suggest that position specific training does not occur in amateur rugby league. The poor fitness of non-elite players may be due to a low playing intensity, infrequent matches of short duration and/or an inappropriate training stimulus

Amra M., (1997) conducted study to establish a data base of norms for boy and girls in the U13, U14, U16, UI8 and the U2I age groups on Anthropometric measures, physiological variables and skills tests were performed on subjects selected from the provincial KwaZulu National Junior Hockey teams in South Africa. The tests were done at the beginning and at the end of season. The anthropometric measures included height, weight, percentage body fat and lean body mass; physiological variables included sit-ups, push-ups, sit-and-reach (flexibility), broad jump, winder and bleep tests, and the skills tests comprised a wide range of ball skill tests. As expected, anthropometric changes were observed across the age groups, due to growth. Amongst the older age groups the girls had reached height and weight values comparable to elite female players , but only the boys in the U2I had reached their adult height and were slightly taller than the elite male players. There was no significant difference in the profile between the attack and defence players in the boys, but amongst the girls the defence players tended to be heavier and taller than the attack players. In the physiological and skills tests there was no difference between positional players. In comparison between pre and end season to determine the effectiveness of the training programmes, there was a change in the anthropometric characteristics because of growth. However, the physiological and skill tests revealed no consistent pattern of improvement in the test results from pre season to end season. This study provides the first set of norms for male and female junior hockey players in South Africa. Further studies are required to expand upon and update the data in the current study.

Khanna, et al. (1996) conducted a study to determine the physical and physiological profile of Kabaddi players and the physiological demands of playing a Kabaddi match. Maximum aerobic capacity (VO2max), maximum ventilation (VEmax), O2 pulse, respiratory equivalent (RE), maximum heart rate, and O2 debt were assessed on 16 players. The somatotype of the players was calculated by the Heath and Carter method. Heart rate was monitored during a selection trial match on eight players who represented India in the Asian Games, 1994. From the playing heart rate, oxygen consumption (VO2) was computed through a heart rate VO2 regression equation. Maximum lactate was evaluated from the blood samples collected at the end of the match. The average heart rate and oxygen consumption during the match were 146.5 (SD 9.25) beats min-1 and 2.25(0.59) liter min-1 respectively. During raiding the maximum heart rate attained varied from 162.4(11.3) to 177.4(4.2) beats min-1. Out of 40 min of match played a raider raided on average on 8.13(2.03) occasions. The average time per raid was 20.8(6.26) s. The match heart rate and oxygen consumption was 72.3-83.3% of the maximum heart rate, and 43.5-70.5% of VO2max respectively. Maximum lactate at the end of the match was 6.13(2.53) min-l litre-1. Kabaddi players had the somatotype of 2.68-4.71-1.83, with absolute back strength of 175.0 kg. VO2max and O2 debt were 3.59(0.36) litre min-1 [47.82(3.68) ml kg-1 min-1] and 5.3(1.85) litres (70 ml kg-1) respectively. Kabaddi is an intermittent sport. The rest pause during the game is sufficient for recovery. During raiding the main source of energy is anaerobic.

Sangral (1994) conducted study on motor fitness components as predictor of talent in hockey. Thirty nine (N=39) male students were selected as sample of study. Ten ball shooting rolling for 25 meters and dribble and roll for 20 seconds test were used to evaluate the hockey performance. Motor fitness used to evaluate the hockey performance. Motor fitness test i.e. co-ordination ability, standing broad jump, 30 metre fly start, vertical jump, 10X6 meter shuttle run, sitting ball throw, 800 metre run and 20 metre backward run were used. The analysis if data showed that 10 ball shooting significant relationship with co-ordination ability and backward run for 20 meter. Similarly rolling of 20 metre had significant relationship with standing broad jump, 30 metre fly start, vertical jump, 10X6 metre shuttle run, sitting ball throw, 800 metre run and backward run for 20 metre, dribble and roll for 20 seconds (distance). The regression equation for prediction showed different contribution of motor abilities to hockey performance.

Vaz, L. W. (1994) investigated some of the selected anthropometric characteristics and physical fitness components as predictors of performance in Judo. He found in his study that anthropometric variables namely height, weight, calf – girth, arm girth and ponderal index were related to judo performance in various weight categories, but leg length, arm length, thigh girth and crural ratio were not seen significantly related to Judo performance. Combined contribution of anthropometric and physical fitness variables to judo performance in various weight categories were showing significant relations. Multiple regression analysis indicated that predictions regarding Judo performance, on the basis of anthropometric and physical fitness variables can be made with reasonable degree of accuracy.

Diwarka (1991) conducted a study to investigate the relationship of physical, physiological and motor skill variables to volleyball playing ability and to assess the combined contribution of physical, physiological and motor skill variables to volleyball playing ability. Physical variables include speed, arm length, explosive power, dynamic balance, agility, flexibility, age, height and weight are taken. Physiological variables including pulse rate, systolic blood pressure, dialstolic blood pressure and cardio-vascular endurance were measured. Motor skill variables were volleying, serving, passing and set-up. 100 50 women volleyball players who participated in the inter-college level tournament were taken as subjects.

Uppal and Datta (1988) conducted study on motor fitness components as predictors of hockey performance seventy four male hockey players of different Universities of Indian secured as the subject of the study. The motor fitness component included speed, strength, power, agility, flexibility, dynamic balance and kinesthetic perception trait. Field hockey rating scale secured as the criterion measure to evaluate the playing ability. It was concluded on the basis of results yielded by the study that motor fitness components

39

of speed, grip strength (both right and left hand), agility, balance and kinesthetic perception contribute to hockey playing ability, where as power and flexibility are not significant contributors to hockey performance.

Dureha D. K (1984) conducted a comparative study on selected motor components such as agility, speed, explosive strength and endurance and selected anthropometric variables such as height, weight, leg length, arm length, thigh girth and wrist diameter of offensive and defensive hockey players at college level. Fifty male students of three colleges of Gwalior during the session 1983-84 were the subjects of the study. The 't' test was employed for the statistical analysis of data to compare the offensive and defensive hockey players. It was concluded from the results of the study that there was no significant difference between offensive and defensive hockey players in respect to selected motor components and selected anthropometric variables.

Dutta (1984) conducted study to investigate the relationship of physical, physiological and psychological variable to performance in hockey and to find out the combined contribution of physical/physiological variable to hockey playing ability beside developing a multiple regression equation for the prediction of hockey performance in the study the physical variable included speed, grip strength, power, agility, dynamic balance, flexibility and kinaesthetic perception and in the physiological variable included cardio respiratory endurance, resting pulse rate, reaction time, movement time, response time and body composition and the psychological variable included anxiety and intelligence analyze of data a revealed significant relationship of hockey playing ability to each of the following physical ,physiological and psychological variable speed (r= -0.29) right grip strength (r= 0.29) left grip strength (r= 0.47) agility (= -0.30) balance (r=0.27) and a kinaesthetic perception (r=0.29) cardio respiratory endurance (r=0.30) resting pulse rate (r= -0.48) hand reaction time (r= -0.49) speed of movement (r= -0.58) response time (r= -0.38) and body composition (r= -0.23) and anxiety (r= -0.48) the relationship

40

between standing broad jump, trunk flexibility and intelligence to hockey playing ability were not found to be statistically significant at .05 level of confidence.

Lamba M.K, (1980) conducted study to compare selected physical fitness components and physiological variables of college level offensive and defensive hockey players. Physical fitness components were agility, speed, strength and physiological variables were blood pressure, pulse rate breath holding capacity and cardiovascular endurance. Sixty male students representing four colleges of Gwalior in 1978 - 79 intercollegiate tournaments acted as the subjects of the study. After administering the tests't' ratio was used to statistically analyze the data. Conclusions of the study were: 1) The offensive players are faster and have less resting pulse rate and thus have more cardiovascular endurance than defensive players; 2) the defensive players have more arm and leg strength than offensive players and 3) there is no difference between offensive and defensive players in agility, blood pressure and breath holding capacity.

Randal W. Reid (1978) conducted study to investigate the relationship of flexibility, strength and anthropometric measurements of the lower limbs to the skating speed of hockey players. Subjects were seventeen University hockey players whenever measured for leg and grip strengths, lower limb flexibility, anthropometry of legs and skating speed understanding and flying start conditions with or without sticks over two distances, 40 ft and 25 mts. The strength, flexibility and anthropometric measures were the independent variables while the skating speeds were the dependent variables. The data were analyzed by Pearson Product Moment, Correlation and stepwise regression methods (P < 0.05). The results of the study indicated that flexibility was specific to each joint measured, there was a general strength factor and a general skating body type two of the skating speed tests encompassed many factors of the other six, flexibility was related to strength and anthropometry, strength and anthropometry were related, and flexibility and anthropometry were not related to skating speed. The

41

regression analysis accounted for all of the variance in each dependent variable but the variables entered were different in order and in contributing weight in each analysis. Skating speed was indicated as being specific to the distance and conditions under which it was performed.

Malhotra et al. (1975) on 24 Indian hockey players described that the mean age, height and weight of the players has to be 23.8 years, 172.5 cms. and 62.9 kg respectively. He concluded that the full backs were found to be the tallest followed by half backs, forwards and goalkeepers.

Dolores (1970) conducted study to establish relationship of shoulder flexibility and other selected factors to throwing performance by college women. Thirty five college freshmen were tested on the over-arm throw involving both accuracy and distance throwing. The variables shoulder flexibility, shoulder strength, speed of arm movement, age, height, weight, background, athletic background, and number and sex of children in the family were studied. Variables which proved to have predictive value in relation to accuracy throwing were the average of shoulder strength, speed of arm movement, athletic background, and the group of three physiological factors. Those variables which showed a significant relationship to determine throwing arm shoulder strength and athletic background, shoulder flexibility was not a significant predictor of throwing; shoulder strength was the best physiological variable flexibility Was highly related to strength, either the accuracy of distance test items could have been used and best predictor of throwing was found athletic experience.

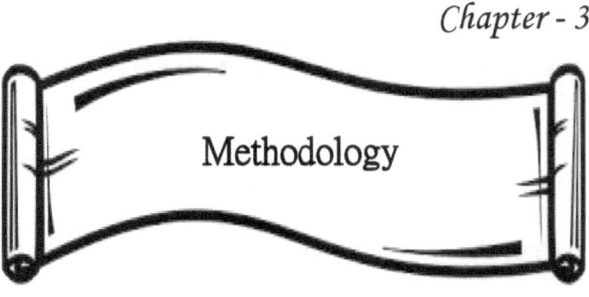

Chapter - 3

Methodology

In this chapter, the selection of subjects, selection of variables, criterion measures, reliability of data, collection of data, administration of the test and statistical techniques which were used for analyzing the data are described.

Selection of Subjects

Sixty male elite field hockey players (30 junior and 30 sub-juniors) were selected for the study. Their age ranged between 17-21 years and14-16 years from junior and sub-junior national tournament and camp. The subjects were selected by random sampling method. All subjects selected for the study were medically and physically fit to take the experimental requirement of this study.

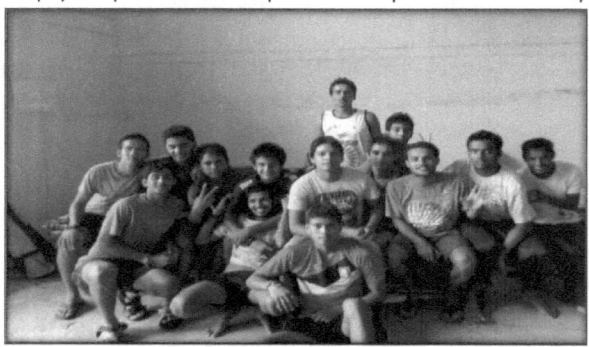

Fig.1: Subjects

Selection of Variables

Through the reviews of literature, with expert's opinion and researcher's own understanding the following variables were selected for the purpose of this study:

- **Anthropometric Variables**
    1. Standing height
    2. Weight
    3. Arm length
    4. Leg length
    5. Thigh girth
    6. Body Fat Percentage
- **Physiological Variables**
    1. Blood pressure
    2. Systolic blood pressure
    3. Diastolic blood pressure
    4. Peak Flow Rate
    5. Resting Heart rate
    6. Aerobic capacity
    7. Body Mass Index (BMI)

Criterion Measures

1. **Standing Height:** - Standing Height was recorded in centimeter with the help of Stadiometer.
2. **Weight:**- Weight was measured in kilogram by used a weighing machine.
3. **Arm length:** - Arm Length was recorded in centimeter with the help of steel tape.
4. **Leg length:** - Leg Length was recorded in centimeter with the help of steel tape.
5. **Thigh girth:** - Thigh Girth was recorded in centimeter with the help of steel tape.

6. Blood pressure: - Blood Pressure was measured in mm/Hg with digital Blood Pressure machine.

7. Peak flow rate: - Peak Flow Rate was recorded in liter/min. with the help of peak flow meter.

8. Resting heart rate: - Resting Heart Rate was recorded number of heart rate per minute during the resting condition.

9. Aerobic capacity: - Aerobic Capacity was recorded in VO_2max (ml/Kg/min) with the help of Cooper 12 min. run and walk test and by using formula of VO_2Max. (Ml/Kg/Min)= (distance covered in meter for 12 minutes run-walk 504.9) / 44.73.

10. Body Mass Index:- Body Mass Index was recorded in kg/m^2 with the help of Height and Weight by using formula of $weight/height^2$

11. Percentage of body fat:- Percentage of Body Fat was obtained by taking Skinfold Measurements at four sites namely biceps, triceps, sub-scapula, and supra-illiac and the total value of four sites was compared to a ready reckoner prapared by Durnin and Rahaman to obtain the percentage of body fat.

Assessment of Performance in Hockey

Performance in Hockey was measured by judging their playing ability. Playing ability of all player were judged (out of 10 points) from a rating scale by a panel of experts and the average of three score was consider as playing ability.

10 Marks- Excellent Performance

8 Marks - Good

6 Marks- Average

4 Marks- Below Average

2 Marks- Poor

Each subject was given marks according to their performance by all 3 judges. From these ratings, the average of three score was taken as performance of the player. This was done to eliminate the chances of biasness among the judges.

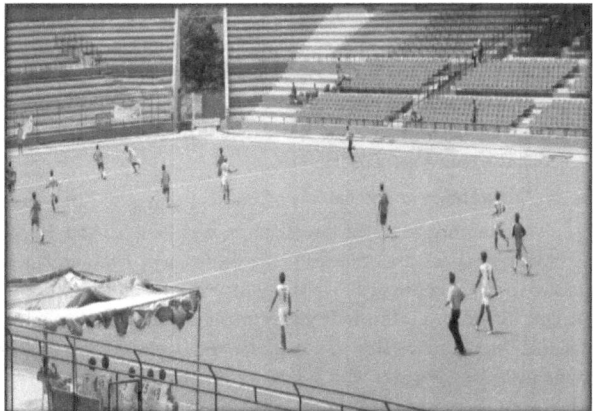

Fig.2: Assessment of Hockey Performance

Collection of Data

The necessary data was collected by administering the tests for the chosen variable. All the test was administered in the hockey field of Sports College of Lucknow and SAI centre Bhopal.

Before the administration of test the subjects were given a chance to practice the prescribed tests so that they became familiar with the tests and knew exactly what was to be done. The use of apparatus was explained to them prior to the administration of tests. To ensure uniform testing condition the subject were tested only during the morning and evening session for anthropometrical and physiological variable respectively.

Reliability of Data

The reliability of data was ensured by establishing the instrument reliability, tester's competency, reliability of test and the subject reliability.

Instrument Reliability

The stop watch, steel tape, digital blood pressure machine, peak flow meter, and skinfold Caliper were used for the test were considered reliable as they were procured from reputed firms and

46

were in use for research purposes. All the instruments used were available in the department of physical education, Banaras Hindu university Varanasi and their calibration were accepted as accurate enough for the purpose of this study. These tests were standard test which had a high reliability and were accompanied by Indian norms, hence, these test were chosen.

Tester Competency and Reliability of Test

To ensure that the investigator was well versed in the technique of conducting the tests, the investigator had number of practice session in the testing procedure under the guidance of Dr. Sushma Ghildyal, professor in department of physical education, Banaras Hindu University Varanasi. All the measurements were taken by the investigator with assistance of other research scholars, who were also well acquainted with the test and their testing procedure. Tester competency was evaluated together with the reliability of test. Reliability of test was established by test retest process whereby consistence of results was obtained by product moment correlation. The data collected from a random selection of a ten subjects in test-retest were computed for each variable and obtain correlation have been shown in table 1.

TABLE-1

Reliability Coefficients of Test, Re-Test Scores

S. No.	Variable	Coefficient of Reliability
1	Standing Height	.99
2	Weight	.97
3	Arm Length	.99
4	Leg Length	.99
5	Thigh Girth	.99
6	Body Fat Percentage	.98
7	Systolic Blood Pressure	.84
8	Diastolic Blood Pressure	.91
9	Resting Heart rate	.87
10	Peak Flow Rate	.73
11	Aerobic Capacity	.85
12	Body Mass Index (BMI)	.97

Subject Reliability

The test and retest co-efficiency of correlation also indicate subject reliability as the same subject were used under similar condition by the same tester. No motivational technique was used at the time of testing.

Orientation of Subjects

In order to get full co-operation from the subject the investigator very clearly explained about the purpose of the study.

Prior to the administration of the test, it was very clearly explained to the subjects in detail about the procedure to be followed during the test. This explanation helped very much to ensure the effectiveness co-operation, from the subject to obtain the reliability of data. Model performance by some of the subjects was also done to make clearly understand the test related to the study.

Administration of Test

The tests were administered with the help of a team of testers and research assistant under the guidance of supervision of the experts. Prior to the administration of the test and equipment the subject was given a chance to practice the prescribed test and equipment so the subject make themselves familiar with the test and equipment and know exactly what has to be done . The use of apparatus was explained to them prior to the administration of the test.

Anthropometric Variables
Standing Height

Purpose: To measures the height of the subject.

Equipment: Wall Scale.

Procedure: The height of the subjects was measured with subject standing erect without shoes, against a wall with a marked scale. The subjects was instructed to keep the heels together, body touching the wall with heels, buttocks and back, head erect without tilt and to take and hold a full breath and stand erect while height measurements are taken. A stiff hard board was held horizontally on his head, slightly pressing the head and touching the scale, marked on the wall, at right angle. The subject was asked to step out by lowering the head and the readings indicated by the lower end of the hard board are taken. Height was recorded to the centimeter.

Weight

Purpose: To measure the weight of the subject

Equipment: Standard weighing machine.

Procedure: Weight of the subjects was taken with the help of a standard and calibrated weighing machine in kilograms. Subjects were asked to come on the weighing machine with short pants. They were asked to stand still keeping the body erect. The scores were recorded to the kilogram.

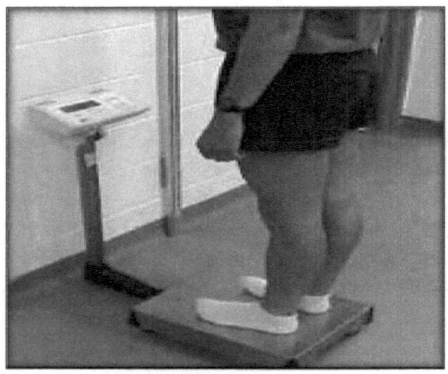

Fig.3: Weight Measurement

Arm Length

Purpose: To Measure the arm Length of the subject.

Equipment: Steel Measuring Tape.

Procedure: Arm length was measured with a flexible steel tape. The subjects were asked to stand erect. Measurement was taken from the acromion process to the tip of the third finger. Measurement was recorded to the nearest centimetre.

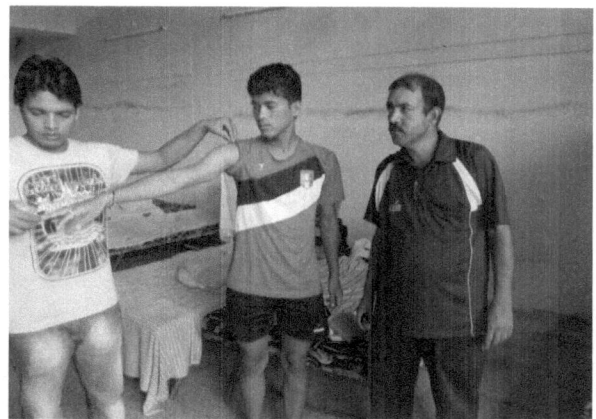

Fig.4: Arm Length Measurement

Leg Length

Purpose: To measure the leg length of the subject

Equipment: Steel Measuring Tape.

Procedure: Leg lengths of the subjects were measured with a flexible steel tape from the bottom outside the edge of the centre of foot to the upper edge of the greater trochanter and are recorded to the nearest centimeter.

Thigh Girth

Purpose: To measure the thigh girth of the subject.

Equipment: Steel measuring tape

Procedure: Thigh girth was measured with a steel tape placed around the thigh horizontally with its top edge under the fold of the buttock. The subject was asked to stand with his weight equally distributed on both feet. It was recorded to the nearest centimeter.

Body Fat Percentage

Purpose: To Measure the Body Fat Percentage of the subject.

Site : Biceps.

Equipment: Lenge's skin fold calliper.

Procedure: The subject was asked to stand at ease with arm hanging at side. Usually the midpoint of the upper arm marked previously for measuring upper arm circumference help to provide land mark for biceps and triceps skin fold. These was also to taken at exactly the same level as of the upper arm circumference .The skin and subcutaneous fat fold was picked at about 1 cm. above the mark level on the anterior side of the biceps muscle. The jaw of the caliper was applied on the fold so that the marked horizontal line was approximately at the level of the midpoint. The jaw holds a double layer of skin plus subcutaneous fat. The lighter arm of the caliper was slowly released so as to pull pressure of the jaw on the vertical skin fold. The reading was noted from the dial of the caliper about 2 sec. after leaving the smaller arm of the caliper. When the reading was quite stable the measurement was recorded in millimetre.

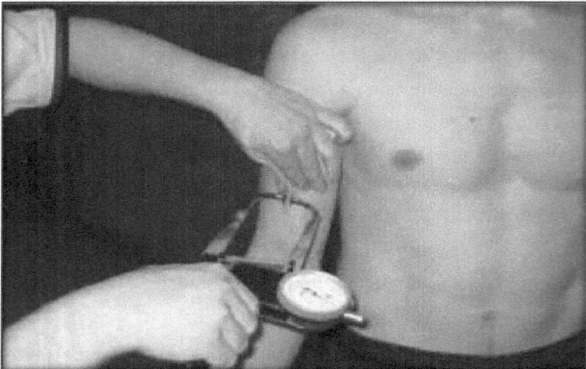

Fig.5: Biceps skinfold Measurement

Site: Triceps

Equipment: Lenge's skin fold caliper

Procedure: The subject was asked to stand at ease with arm hanging at side. The midpoint of the upper arm marked previously for measuring upper arm circumference help to provide land mark for measuring triceps skinfold. The skin and subcutaneous fat fold was

51

picked at about 1 cm. above the mark level on the posterior side of the triceps muscle. The jaw of the caliper applied on the fold, so that the marked horizontal line was approximately at the level of the midpoint of the jaw and the jaw holds a double layer of skin plus subcutaneous fat. The lighter arm of the caliper was slowly released so as to put full pressure of the jaw on the vertical skin fold. The reading was noted from the dial of the caliper about 2 sec. after leaving. When the reading was quite stable the measurement was recorded in millimetre.

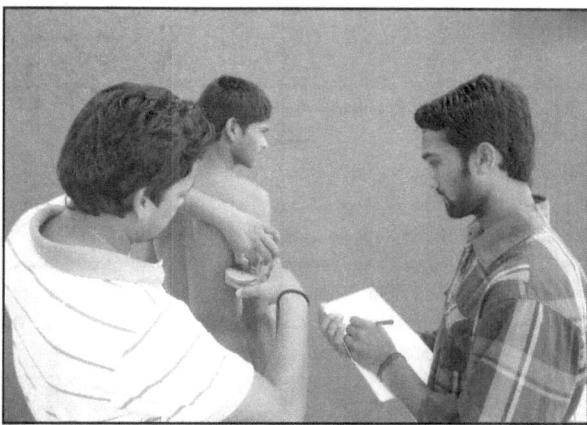

Fig.6: Triceps skinfold Measurement

Site: Subscapular

Equipment: Lenge's skin fold caliper

Procedure: The tester picked skinfold diagonally below the anterior angle of the scapula almost parallel to medial border of scapula in such a way that the skinfold from an angle of roughly 45° to the horizontal, with its lower and pointing outwards. The jaw of caliper was applied about a millimetre below the fold picking tip of thumb. The measurement as usually was record after two second of releasing full pressure on the fold.

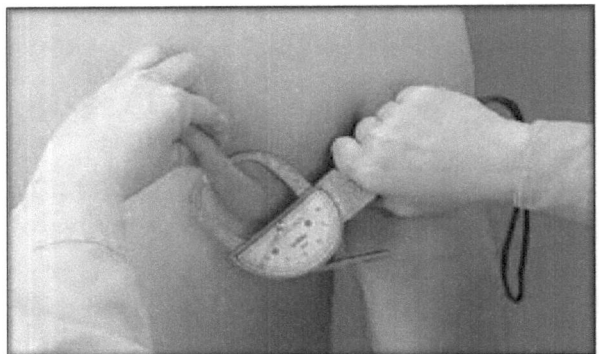

Fig.7: Subscapula skinfold Measurement

Site: Suprailiac

Equipment: Lenge's skin fold caliper

Procedure: The subject skinfold was lifted about 1 cm. above 2 cm. medial to the anterior superior iliac spine of the left side. The jaw of the skinfold caliper was applied parallel to the natural direction of the picked up skin fold. This was usually horizontal or slightly oblique pointing upward and latterly downwards medially. The reading was recorded in millimetre.

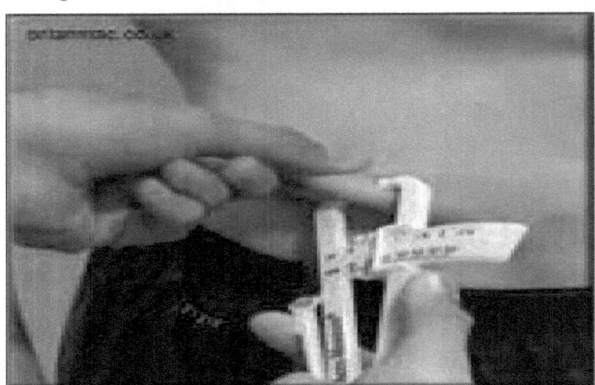

Fig.8: Supra-iliac skinfold Measurement

53

Scoring: The measurement was recorded to the nearest millimetre. The sum of the skinfold thickness of four sites of the body was converted into percentage of body fat with the help of the standard table suggested by Durnin and Rahaman.

Physiological Variables

Resting Heart Rate

Purpose: To measure the resting heart rate of the subjects.

Equipment: Stop watch

Procedure: Heart rate was obtained in early morning by the scholar, subject were approached in the rooms of the hostel where they were stay. A calibrated stop watch and a stethoscope was used for counting heart rate. The subjects was requested not to leave their bed and in case somebody moved out he as requested to lie down quietly for ten minutes before taking his heart rate. Total number of heart beats per minute for each subject was recorded as his score.

Blood Pressure

Purpose: To measure the diastolic and systolic blood pressure of the subject

Equipment: Mercury sphygmomanometer, cuff, and stethoscope.

Procedure: The sphygmomanometer was placed on a bench where the subject could not see the mercury column. Blood pressure was recorded after the subject has rested quietly for 5 minutes, and this measure should precede all other measures. The subject was seated with the arm resting on the bench, the elbow approximately at the level of the heart. The cuff was attached, the pressure then increased to approximately 180 mm Hg. The stethoscope will placed over the brachial artery in the cubital fossa. The pressure was released at a rate of approximately 2 mm per second. The pressure at which the first sounds was heard (systolic pressure) and the pressure when all sounds disappear (diastolic pressure) was recorded.

Measurement: Blood pressure was recorded in the units of millimetres of mercury (mm/ Hg).

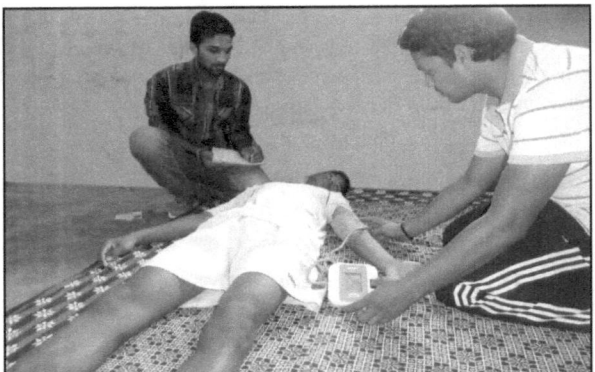

Fig.9: Blood Pressure Measurement

Peak Flow Rate

Purpose: To measure the rate of flow of air per minute of the peak expiratory condition

Equipment: Peak flow meter, electronic digital watch.

Procedure: The subject was asked to take a deep breath and blow it into the mouthpiece of peak flow meter as forcefully as possible and maintain steadily for a few second to take the reading. The level to each the indicator rises was read ard recorded in litre/minutes.

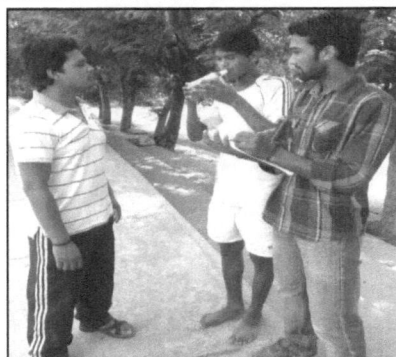

Fig.10: Peak Flow Measurement

Body Mass Index (BMI)

Purpose: To measure body mass index of the subjects.

Equipment: Steel tape, weighing machine

Procedure: Body Mass Index (BMI) is a Weight-to-Height ratio which is calculated by dividing the body weight in kilograms by the height in meters squared (kg/m^2). The height and weight measurement were put in following formula to calculate BMI.

$$BMI = Weight, (kg) / Height, (m)^2$$

Aerobic Capacity

Purpose: To measure the aerobic capacity

Equipment: 400mts. Standard track, marking for the test, whistle and stopwatch.

Procedure: The subjects were divided in two groups and partner of each student was assigned. While one student was running, the partner was instructed to count the number of laps that his partner had covered within the allotted time.

Scoring: The number of laps and extra covered distance in Meter was recorded as the score of the subject.

$VO_2Max.$ (Ml/Kg/Min)= (distance covered in meter for 12 minutes run-walk 504.9) / 44.73

Statistical Techniques Employed for Analysis

To assess the performance on the basis of selected anthropometric and physiological variables of Junior and Sub junior Field hockey players following statistical technique was applied-

1. To characterize the anthropometric and physiological variables of Junior and Sub junior Field hockey players, descriptive statistic was used.

2. To find out relationship between dependent variable (Hockey performance) and independent variables (anthropometric and physiological variables), Pearson's Product Moment method of correlation was used.

3. To find out joint contribution of independent variables (selected anthropometric and physiological variables) in

56

predicting dependent variable (Hockey performance), Multiple Correlation was used.

4. For predicting dependent variable (Hockey performance) on the basis of independent variables (anthropometric and physiological variables), Multiple regression equation was established.

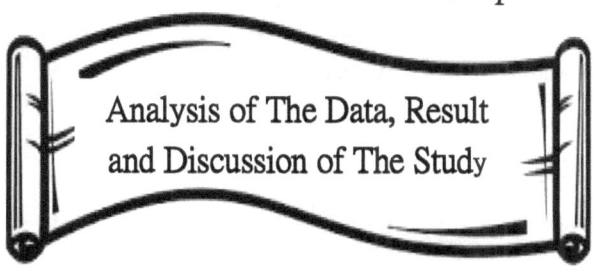

Chapter - 4

Analysis of The Data, Result and Discussion of The Study

The statistical analysis of data has been presented in this chapter. The Anthropometric variables namely Standing Height, Weight, Arm Length, Leg Length Thigh Girth, percentage of body fat and Physiological Variables namely Blood Pressure, Resting Heart rate, Peak flow rate, BMI (Body mass Index), Aerobic capacity were collected on 60 male Hockey players, 30 in each category i.e. Sub – Junior, Junior.

Level of Significance

The level of significance was set at 0.05 levels which were considered appropriate for the purpose of the study.

Findings

The findings with regard to the present study have been presented in two sections.

Section - 1

To study of Physiological variables, Anthropometric variables and Performance of Sub Junior and Junior Hockey Players, descriptive statistics were computed and data pertaining to that is presented in TABLE – 2 to 7.

TABLE-2

Descriptive Analysis of Selected Anthropometric Variables of Sub-Junior Hockey Players (N=30)

Variables	Mean	S.D	Variance	Skew.	Kurt.	Range	Min.	Max.	SE
Height	164.13	6.40	40.95	-.85	.26	24.00	150.00	174.00	1.17
Weight	54.57	6.46	41.77	.35	.56	31.00	41.00	72.00	1.18
Arm Length	74.01	2.49	6.20	-.76	-.05	8.80	68.70	77.50	.45
Leg Length	98.33	4.21	17.75	-.35	-.01	18.00	89.00	107.00	.77
Thigh Girth	48.80	3.28	10.79	.67	.52	14.00	43.00	57.00	.60
Body Fat Percentage	13.45	1.93	3.72	.32	.86	8.20	9.70	17.90	.35

Table-2 revealed that the average values of anthropometrical variable of sub-junior Hockey players were: Height 164.13±6.40, Weight 54.57±6.46, Arm Length 74.01±2.49, Leg Length 98.33±4.21, Thigh Girth 48.80±3.28 and Percentage of body fat 13.45±.1.93.

In the same categories, the minimum and maximum values for anthropometric variables were: Height (150.00; 174.00), Weight (41.00; 72.00), Arm Length (68.70; 77.50), Leg Length (89.00; 107.00), Thigh Girth (43.00; 57.00) and Percentage of body fat (9.70; 17.90).

The variables like Height, Arm Length and Leg Length were negatively skewed, where as variable like Weight, Thigh Girth, Percentage of body fat were positively skewed. Negatively skewed distribution shows that most of the data is on higher side whereas positively skewed distribution shows that most of the data is on lower side.

The value of kurtosis like Arm Length, Leg Length was negative whereas Height, Weight, Thigh Girth, Percentage of body fat was positive. Negative kurtosis shows that data on these variables was more variable than that of normal distribution whereas positive kurtosis shows that data on these variables was less variable than that of normal distribution. On looking at the value of coefficient of variance it was found that the maximum variability was 41.77 in relation to weight whereas minimum variability was 3.72 in percentage of body fat.

TABLE-3
Descriptive Analysis of Selected Physiological Variables of Sub-Junior Hockey Players (N=30)

Variables	Mean	S.D	Variance	Skew.	Kurt.	Range	Min.	Max.	SE
Systolic Blood Pressure	119.07	6.66	44.41	-.29	1.66	33.00	102.00	135.00	1.22
Diastolic Blood Pressure	70.20	4.52	20.44	-.50	1.26	21.00	57.00	78.00	.83
Resting Heart Rate	56.47	5.91	34.88	-.09	-.45	23.00	43.00	66.00	1.08
Peak Flow Rate	406.67	48.52	2354.02	-.47	-.88	160.00	320.00	480.00	8.86
Aerobic Capacity	42.12	5.86	34.30	-1.76	1.18	28.61	20.46	49.07	1.07
Body Mass Index	20.20	1.39	1.94	.64	.24	6.03	17.75	23.78	.25

Table-3 revealed that the average values of physiological variables of sub-junior Hockey players were: Systolic Blood Pressure 119.07±6.66, Diastolic Blood Pressure 70.20±4.52 Resting Heart Rate 56.47±5.91, Peak flow rate 406.67±48.52 Aerobic capacity 42.12±5.86 and Body mass index 20.20±1.39.

In the same categories, the minimum and maximum values for physiological variables were: Systolic Blood Pressure (102.00; 135.00), Diastolic Blood Pressure (57.00; 78.00) Resting Heart Rate

(43.00; 66.00), Peak flow rate (320.00; 480.00), Aerobic capacity (20.46; 49.07) and Body mass index (17.75; 23.78).

The variables like Systolic Blood Pressure, Diastolic Blood Pressure, Resting Heart Rate, Peak flow rate, Aerobic capacity were negatively skewed, where as variable like Body mass index were positively skewed. Negatively skewed distribution shows that most of the data is on higher side whereas positively skewed distribution shows that most of the data is on lower side.

Since the value of kurtosis like Resting Heart Rate, Peak flow rate were negative whereas Systolic Blood Pressure, Diastolic Blood Pressure, Aerobic capacity, Body mass index were positive. Negative kurtosis shows that data on these variables was more variable than that of normal distribution whereas positive kurtosis shows that data on these variables was less variable than that of normal distribution. On looking at the value of coefficient of variance it was found that the maximum variability was 2354.02 in relation to Peak flow rate whereas minimum variability was 1.94 in Body mass index.

TABLE-4
Descriptive Analysis of Performance of Sub-Junior Hockey Players (N=30)

	Mean	S.D	Variance	Skew.	Kurt.	Range	Min.	Max.	SE
Performance	7.79	1.03	1.07	-.44	-.59	4.00	5.33	9.33	.19

Table-4 revealed that the average values of Performance of sub-junior Hockey players were: 7.78±1.03. In the same minimum and maximum values is (5.33; 9.33). Performance was negatively skewed, it shows that most of the score is on higher side. The value of kurtosis was also negative and it shows that data on these variables were more variable than that of normal distribution. On looking at the value of coefficient of variance it was found the variability was 1.07 in relation to performance.

61

TABLE-5

Descriptive Analysis of Selected Anthropometric Variables of
Junior Hockey Players (N=30)

Variables	Mean	S.D	Variance	Skew.	Kurt.	Range	Min.	Max.	SE
Height	170.73	5.39	29.10	1.12	1.26	22.00	163.00	185.00	.98
Weight	61.10	4.99	24.85	-.14	-.75	20.00	50.00	70.00	.91
Arm Length	76.59	1.94	3.75	.38	.32	7.80	73.20	81.00	.35
Leg Length	100.53	4.38	19.19	.68	.12	19.00	92.00	111.00	.80
Thigh Girth	48.25	2.56	6.53	.51	-.75	8.50	45.00	53.50	.47
Body Fat Percentage	12.91	2.31	5.34	.38	-.40	8.30	9.00	17.30	.42

Table-5 revealed that average value of anthropometrical variable of junior Hockey players were: Height 170.73±5.39, Weight 61.10±4.98, Leg Length 100.53±4.38, Arm Length 76.59±1.93, Thigh Girth 48.25±2.31 and Percentage of body fat 12.91±.2.31.

In the same categories, the minimum and maximum values for anthropometric variables were: Height (163.00; 185.00), Weight (50.00; 70.00), Arm Length (73.20; 81.00), Leg Length (92.00; 111.00), Thigh Girth (45.00; 53.50) and Percentage of body fat (9.00; 17.30).

The variables like Weight was negatively skewed, where as variable like Height, Arm Length, Leg Length, Thigh Girth, Percentage of body fat were positively skewed. Negatively skewed distribution shows that most of the data is on higher side whereas positively skewed distribution shows that most of the data is on lower side.

The value of kurtosis like Weight, Thigh Girth, Percentage of body fat were negative whereas Height, Arm Length, Leg Length were positive. Negative kurtosis shows that data on these variables was more variable than that of normal distribution whereas positive kurtosis shows that data on these variables was less variable than that of normal distribution. On looking at the value of coefficient of variance it was found that the maximum variability was 29.10 in relation to Height whereas minimum variability was 3.75 in Arm Length.

<u>**TABLE-6**</u>

Descriptive Analysis of Selected Physiological Variables of Junior Hockey Players (N=30)

Variables	Mean	S.D	Variance	Skew.	Kurt.	Range	Min.	Max.	SE
Systolic Blood Pressure	122.30	6.04	36.42	.24	-.46	25.00	110.00	135.00	1.10
Diastolic Blood Pressure	64.10	5.52	30.44	-.61	.77	24.00	51.00	75.00	1.01
Resting Heart Rate	64.67	4.44	19.68	-.52	.00	17.00	55.00	72.00	72.00
Peak Flow Rate	506.00	53.92	2907.59	.20	-1.27	170.00	420.00	590.00	9.84
Aerobic Capacity	50.82	5.85	34.28	1.03	1.26	22.35	43.49	65.84	65.84
Body Mass Index	20.95	1.29	1.68	.80	-.17	4.99	18.82	23.81	.24

Table-6 revealed that average value of physiological variables of junior Hockey players were: Systolic Blood Pressure 122.30±6.03, Diastolic Blood Pressure 64.10±5.52 Resting Heart Rate 64.67±4.44, Peak flow rate 506.00±53.92 Aerobic capacity 50.81±5.85 and Body mass index 20.95±1.29.

In the same categories, the minimum and maximum values for physiological variables were: Systolic Blood Pressure (110.00; 135.00), Diastolic Blood Pressure (51.00; 75.00) Resting Heart Rate (55.00; 72.00), Peak flow rate (420.00; 590.00), Aerobic capacity (43.49; 65.84) and Body mass index (18.82; 23.81).

The variables like Diastolic Blood Pressure, Resting Heart Rate, were negatively skewed where as variable like Systolic Blood Pressure, Peak flow rate, Aerobic capacity Body mass index were positively skewed. Negatively skewed distribution shows that most of the data is on higher side whereas positively skewed distribution shows that most of the data is on lower side.

The value of kurtosis like Systolic Blood Pressure, Peak flow rate, Body mass index were negative whereas Diastolic Blood Pressure, Resting Heart Rate, Aerobic capacity were positive. Negative kurtosis shows that data on these variables was more variable than that of normal distribution whereas positive kurtosis shows that data on these variables was less variable than that of normal distribution. On looking at the value of coefficient of variance it was found that the maximum variability was 2907.59 in relation to Peak flow rate whereas minimum variability was 1.68 in Body mass index.

TABLE-7

Descriptive Analysis of Performance of Junior Hockey Players (N=30)

	Mean	S.D	Variance	Skew.	Kurt.	Range	Min.	Max.	SE
Performance	7.83	1.29	1.66	-.73	.44	5.34	4.66	10.00	.24

Table-7 revealed that average value of Performance of junior Hockey players were: 7.83±1.29. In the same minimum and maximum values is (4.66; 10.00). Performance was negatively skewed it shows that most of the score is on higher side. Since the value of kurtosis was positive it shows that data on these variables was less variable than that of normal distribution. On looking at the value of coefficient of variance it was found the variability was 1.66 in relation to performance.

Section – 2

To determine the relationship of Physiological and Anthropometric variables with the Hockey Performance, the data collected was analyzed using the correlation (Pearson Product Moment Correlation). Moreover, Regression equation was established by using SPSS version 20 and results pertaining to that have been presented in tables 8 to 23.

TABLE – 8

Relationship between Dependent Variable (Hockey Performance) and Independent Variables (Selected Anthropometric variables) of Sub-Junior Hockey Players

Independent Variables	Correlation coefficient
Height	.000
Weight	-.469*
Arm Length	-.036
Leg Length	-.015
Thigh Girth	-.256
Percentage of Body Fat	-.679*

*Significant at .05 level

$r_{0.05}(28) = 0.361$

Table -8 revealed that Hockey Performance was found significantly correlated with Weight and Percentage of body fat as the correlation coefficient values (-.469, -.679) were found higher than the tabulated value at 0.05 level of significance. Hockey Performance was found not significantly with Height, Arm length, Leg length, and Thigh Girth as the correlation coefficient values were found lower than the tabulated value at 0.05 level of significance.

TABLE-9

Joint Contribution of Independent Variables (Selected
Anthropometric variables) in Predicting Dependent Variable
(Hockey Performance) of Sub-Junior Hockey Players

Criterion Variables	Independent variables	Coefficient of Multiple Correlation
Hockey Performance	Height	.914*
	Weight	
	Arm Length	
	Leg Length	
	Thigh Girth	
	Percentage of body fat	

* Significant at .05 level.

$r_{0.05}$ (23) = 0.396

Table-9 indicates significant relationship between criterion
variable (Hockey Performance) and independent variables (Selected
Anthropometric variable) as coefficient of multiple correlations
0.914 is higher than the tabulated value at 0.05 level of significance.

TABLE-10

Model Summary

R Square	Adjusted R Square	Standard Error
.836	.793	.470

The above table 10 shows that Adjusted R Square (.793) as
predictor was included, which means that 79.3% of the variance in
the performance of Hockey player was associated with changes in
the Anthropometric variables.

TABLE-11

Analysis of Variance for the Regression

	Sum of Square	df	Mean Square	F	Significant
Regression	25.89	6	4.32		
Residual	5.09	23	.22	19.51*	.000
Total	30.98	29	4.54		

* Significant at .05 level

$F_{0.05}$ **(6, 23) =2.53**

Finding of table 11 revealed that developed regression model is significant for prediction of criterion variable and model can be used for further prediction, as value of 'F'(19.51) was found significant at 0.05 level of significance.

TABLE-12

Coefficients[a]

Model	Unstandardized Coefficients		Standardized Coefficients	t	Sig.
	B	Std. Error	Beta		
(Constant)	-8.103	4.694		-1.726	.098
ARM LENGTH	-.304	.140	-.731	-2.163	.041
LEG LENGTH	-.071	.036	-.290	-1.958	.063
THIGH GIRTH	.075	.042	.238	1.785	.087
HEIGHT	.344	.062	2.129	5.523	.000
WEIGHT	-.236	.043	-1.474	-5.465	.000
FAT	-.138	.071	-.258	-1.945	.064

a. Dependent Variable:

The above table displayed the value of the coefficient in the regression equation and measures the probability that a linear relationship existed between anthropometric variable and hockey performance. In this table 'B' was the slope of the line. 'SE B' was the standard error of 'B'. 'Beta' was the standardized regression coefficient. 'Sig' was the significance level for the test of the null hypothesis that the value of a coefficient was zero in the population.

Estimation of Hockey Performance on the basis of selected Anthropometric variables of Sub-Junior Hockey Players

Multiple Regression Analysis

The multiple regression equation for predicting the Hockey Performance on the basis of relative contribution of six anthropometric variables of Sub-junior group resulted in the following-

Equation-1

$$Y= -8.103+0.344 (X_1) -0.236(X_2) -0.304(X_3)-0.071(X_4) +0.075(X_5) -0.138 (X_6)$$

Y=Predictor (Hockey Performance)

X_1=Height

X_2= Weight

X_3= Arm Length

X4= Leg Length

X_5=Thigh Girth

X_6=Percentage of Body Fat

The above mentioned regression equation shows that Hockey Performance depend upon the Height, weight, Arm length, Leg Length, Thigh Girth and Percentage of body fat.

Relationship between Hockey Performance and Anthropometric Variable of Sub-Junior Hockey Player are presented in Figure 13 to 18 and combined relationship between Hockey Performance and Selected Anthropometric Variable of Sub-Junior Hockey Player is shown in Figure 19.

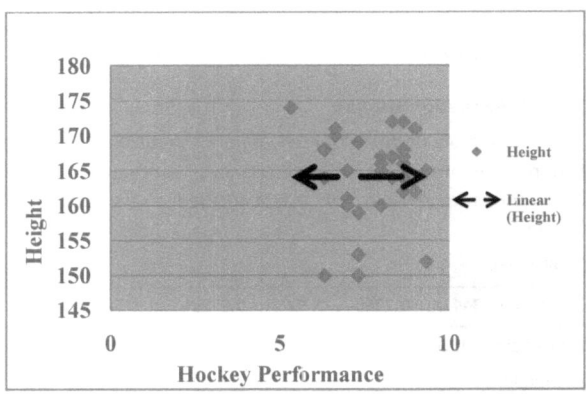

Figure-11: Relationship between Hockey Performance and Height of Sub-Junior Hockey Players

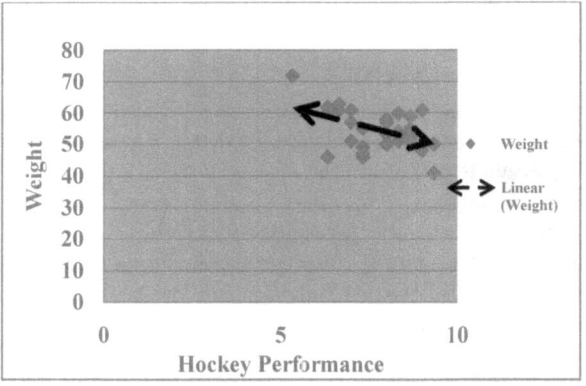

Figure-12: Relationship between Hockey Performance and Weight of Sub-Junior Hockey Players

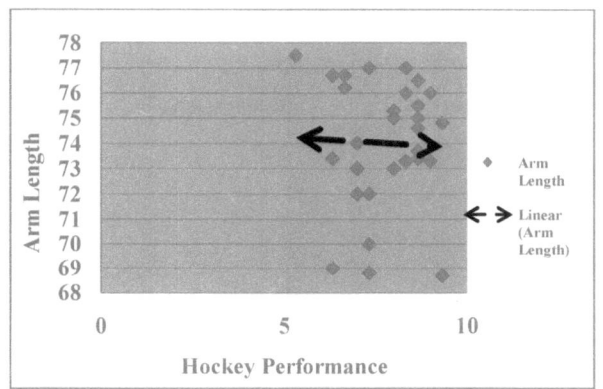

Figure-13: Relationship between Hockey Performance and Arm Length of Sub-Junior Hockey Players

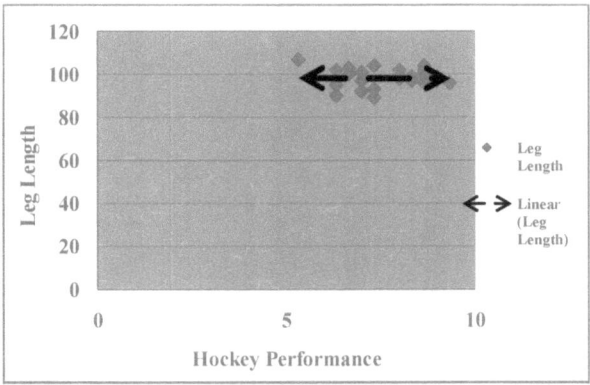

Figure-14: Relationship between Hockey Performance and Leg Length of Sub-Junior Hockey Players

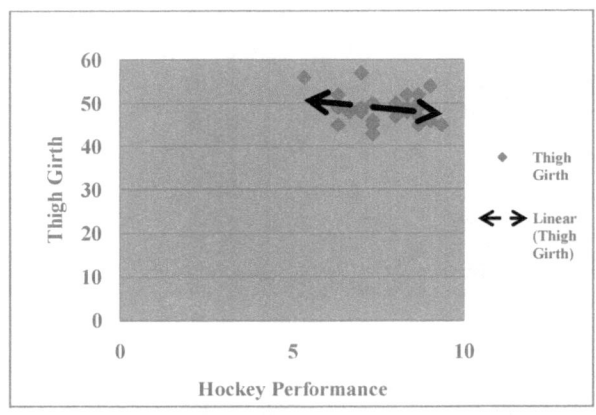

Figure-15: Relationship between Hockey Performance and Thigh Girth of Sub-Junior Hockey Players

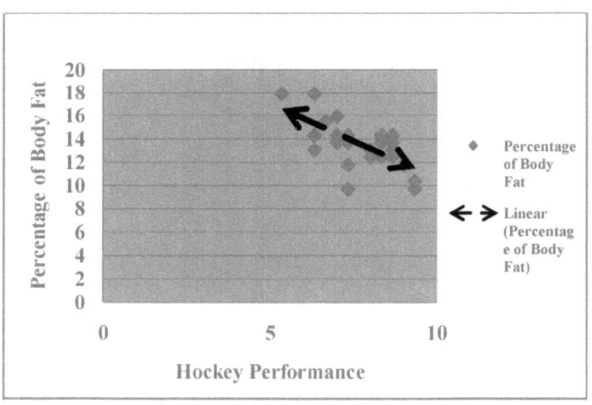

Figure-16: Relationship between Hockey Performance and Percentage of Body Fat of Sub-Junior Hockey Players

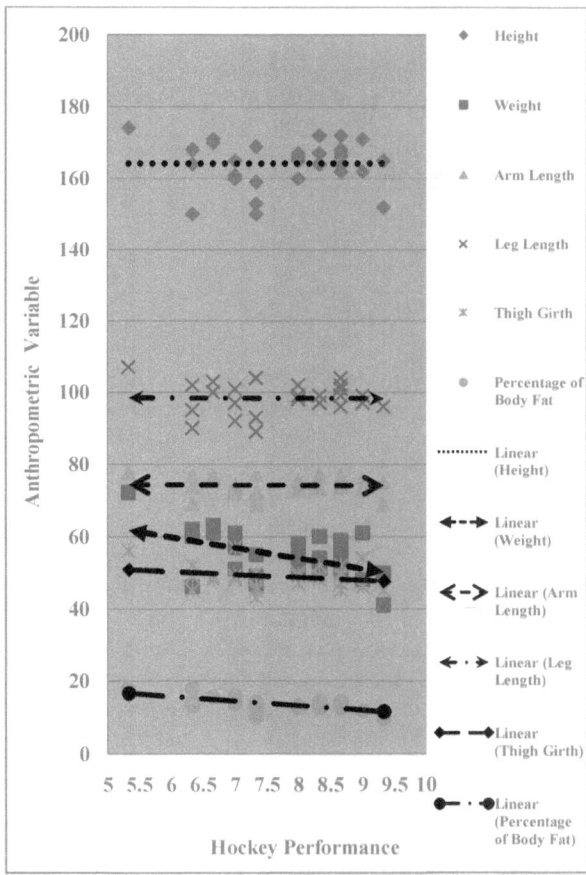

Figure-17: Combined Relationship between Dependent Variable (Hockey Performance) and Independent Variable (Selected Anthropometric Variable) of Sub- Junior Hockey Players

TABLE – 13

Relationship between Dependent Variable (Hockey Performance) and Independent Variables (Selected Anthropometric variables) of Junior Hockey Players

Independent Variables	Correlation coefficient
Height	.032
Weight	-.453*
Arm Length	-.011
Leg Length	.022
Thigh Girth	-.159
Percentage of body fat	-.796*

*Significant at .05 level

$r_{0.05}(28) = 0.361$

Table -12 revealed that Hockey performance was found significantly correlated with Weight and Percentage of body fat as the correlation coefficient values (-.453, -.796) were found higher than the tabulated value at 0.05 level of significance, while Hockey Performance was found not significant with Height, Arm length, Leg length, and Thigh Girth as the correlation coefficient values were found Lower than the tabulated value at 0.05 level of significance.

TABLE – 14

Joint Contribution of Independent Variables (Selected Anthropometric Variables) in Predicting Dependent Variable (Hockey Performance) of Junior Hockey Players

Criterion Variables	Independent variables	Coefficient of multiple correlation
Hockey Performance	Height	.888*
	Weight	
	Arm Length	
	Leg Length	
	Thigh Girth	
	Percentage of body fat	

* Significant at .05 level.

$r_{0.05}(23) = 0.396$

Table-13 indicates significant relationship between criterion variables *(Hockey Performance)* and independent variables *(Selected Anthropometric Characteristics)* as coefficient of multiple correlations was found .888 which is higher than the tabulated value.

TABLE – 15

Model Summary

R Square	Adjusted R Square	Standard Error
.789	.745	.651

The above table 14 shows that Adjusted R Square (.745) as predictor was included, which means that 74.5% of the variance in the performance of Hockey player was associated with changes in the Anthropometric variable.

TABLE – 16

Analysis of Variance for the Regression

	Sum of Square	df	Mean Square	F	Significant
Regression	38.02	5	7.61		
Residual	10.18	24	.42	17.93*	.000
Total	48.20	29			

* Significant at .05 level

$F_{0.05}$ (5, 24) =2.51

Finding of table 15 revealed that developed regression model is significant for prediction of criterion variable and model can be used for further prediction, as value of 'F' (17.93) was found significant at 0.05 level of significance.

TABLE – 17

Coefficients[a]

Model	Unstandardized Coefficients		Standardized Coefficients	t	Sig.
	B	Std. Error	Beta		
(Constant)	21.809	6.680		3.265	.003
ARMLENGTH	-.327	.165	-.490	-1.982	.059
LEGLENGTH	-.129	.055	-.439	-2.347	.028
HEIGHT	.202	.074	.844	2.724	.012
WEIGHT	-.077	.042	-.298	-1.846	.077
FAT	-.442	.070	-.792	-6.288	.000

a. Dependent Variable:

The above table displayed the value of the coefficient in the regression equation and measures the probability that a linear relationship existed between Anthropometric variables and the Hockey Performance. In this table 'B' was the slope of the line. 'SE B' was the standard error of 'B'. 'Beta' was the standardized regression coefficient. 'Sig' was the significance level for the test of the null hypothesis that the value of a coefficient was zero in the population.

Estimation of Hockey Performance on the basis of selected Anthropometric variables of Junior Hockey Players

Multiple Regression Analysis

The multiple regression equation for predicting the Hockey Performance on the basis of relative contribution of five anthropometric variables of junior group resulted in the following-

Equation-2

$$Y = 21.809 + 0.202 (X_1) - 0.077 (X_2) - .327 (X_3) - 0.129 (X_4) - 0.442 (X_6)$$

Y=Predictor (Hockey Performance)

X_1=Height

X_2= Weight

X_3= Arm Length

X_4= Leg Length

X_6=Percentage of Body Fat

The above mentioned regression equation shows that Hockey Performance depend upon the Height, weight, Arm length, Leg Length and Percentage of body fat.

Relationship between Hockey Performance and Anthropometric Variable of Junior Hockey Player are presented in Figure 20 to 25 and combined relationship between Hockey Performance and Selected Anthropometric Variable of Junior Hockey Player is shown in Figure 26.

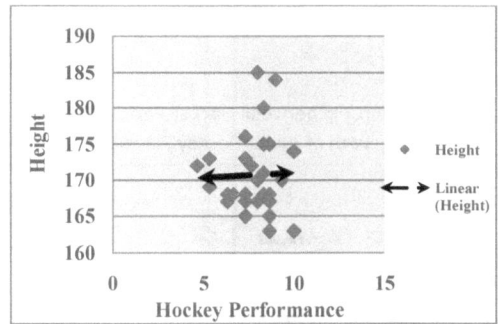

Figure-18: Relationship between Hockey Performance and Height of Junior Hockey Players

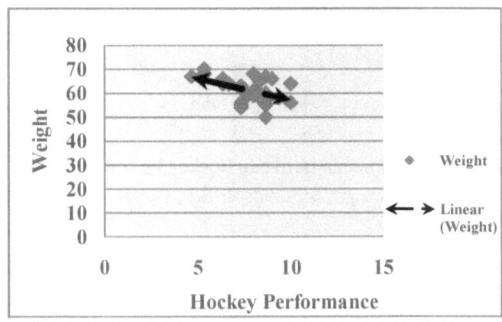

Figure-19: Relationship between Hockey Performance and Weight of Junior Hockey Players

76

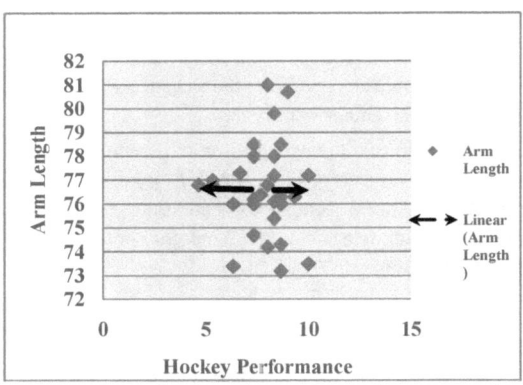

Figure-20: Relationship between Hockey Performance and Arm
Length of Junior Hockey Players

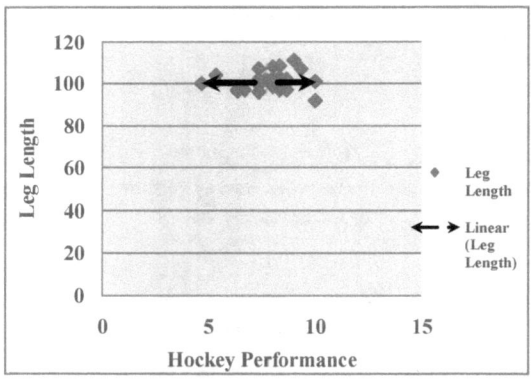

Figure-21: Relationship between Hockey Performance and Leg
Length of Junior Hockey Player

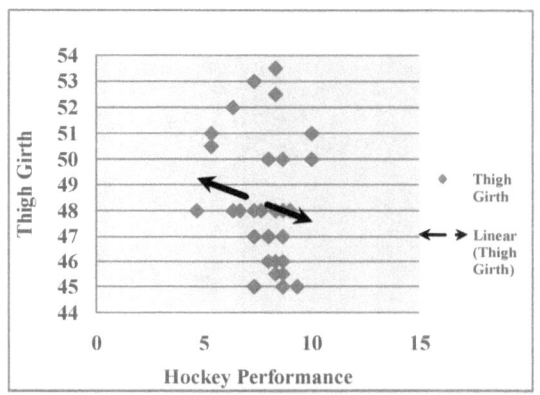

Figure-22: Relationship between Hockey Performance and Thigh Girth of Junior Hockey Players

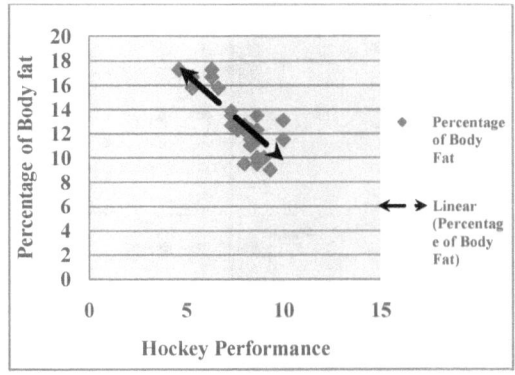

Figure-23: Relationship between Hockey Performance and Percentage of Body fat of Junior Hockey Players

78

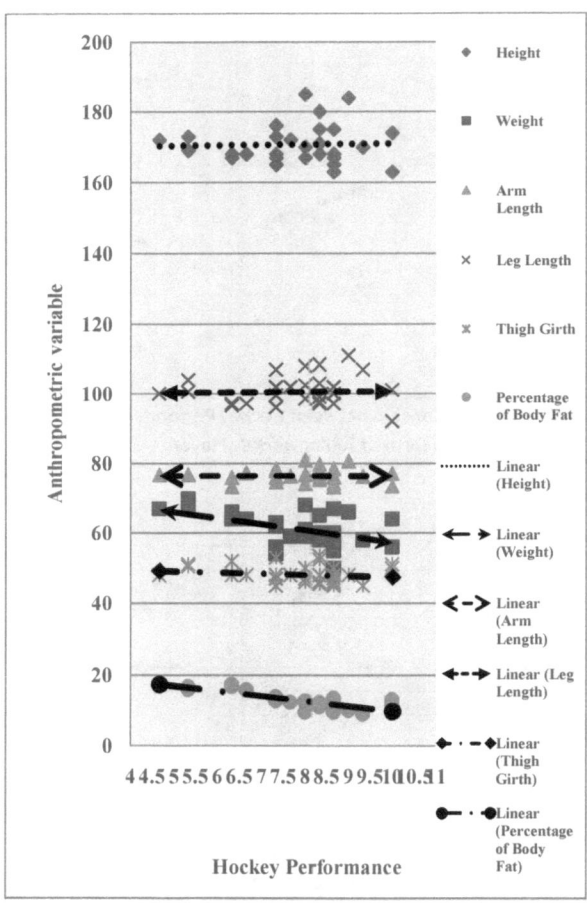

Figure-24: Combined Relationship between Dependent Variable
(Hockey Performance) and Independent Variable (Selected
Anthropometric Variable) of Junior Hockey Players

TABLE – 18

Relationship between Dependent Variable (Hockey Performance) and Independent Variables (Selected Physiological variables) of Sub-Junior Hockey Players

Independent Variables	Correlation coefficient
Systolic Blood Pressure	-.036
Diastolic Blood Pressure	-.104
Resting Heart rate	-.463*
Peak flow rate	.621*
Aerobic capacity	.559*
Body mass index	-.783*

*Significant at .05 level

$r_{0.05}(28) = 0.361$

Table -16 revealed that Hockey performance was found significantly correlated with Resting Heart rate, Peak flow rate, Aerobic capacity, Body mass index as the correlation coefficient values (-.463, .621, .559, -.783) were found higher than the tabulated value at 0.05 level of significance, while Hockey Performance was found not significant with Systolic Blood Pressure, Diastolic Blood Pressure as the correlation coefficient values were found lower than the tabulated value at 0.05 level of significance.

TABLE – 19

Joint Contribution of Independent Variables (Selected Physiological variables) in Predicting Dependent Variable (Hockey Performance) of Sub-Junior Hockey Players

Criterion Variables	Independent variables	Coefficient of multiple correlation
Hockey Performance	Systolic Blood Pressure	.891*
	Diastolic Blood Pressure	
	Resting Heart rate	
	Peak flow rate	
	Aerobic capacity	
	Body mass index	

* Significant at .05 level.

$r_{0.05}(23) = 0.396$

Table-17 indicates significant relationship between criterion variables (Hockey Performance) and independent variables (Selected physiological Characteristics) as coefficient of multiple correlations was found 0.891 which is higher than the tabulated value.

TABLE – 20

Model Summary

R Square	Adjusted R Square	Standard Error
.793	.750	.517

The above table 18 shows that Adjusted R Square (.750) as predictor was included, which means that 75% of the variance in the performance of Hockey player was associated with changes in the physiological variable.

TABLE – 21

Analysis of Variance for the Regression

	Sum of Square	df	Mean Square	F	Significant
Regression	24.57	5	4.91		
Residual	6.41	24	.27	18.40*	.000
Total	30.98	29			

* Significant at .05 level

$F_{0.05} (5, 24) = 2.51$

Finding of table 19 revealed that developed regression model is significant for prediction of criterion variable and model can be used for further prediction, as value of 'F' (18.40) was found significant at 0.05 level of significance.

TABLE – 22

Coefficients[a]

Model	Unstandardized Coefficients		Standardized Coefficients	t	Sig.
	B	Std. Error	Beta		
(Constant)	16.430	2.998		5.481	.000
DIASTOLIC B P	-.037	.021	-.160	-1.721	.098
RESTING EART RATE	-.031	.018	-.179	-1.758	.091
PEAK FLOW RATE	.005	.002	.221	1.980	.059
AEROBIC CAPACITY	.043	.018	.245	2.372	.026
BODY MASS INDEX	-.398	.082	-.536	-4.846	.000

a. Dependent Variable:

The above table displayed the value of the coefficient in the regression equation and measures the probability that a linear relationship existed between physiological variables and the Hockey Performance. In this table 'B' was the slope of the line. 'SE B' was the standard error of 'B'. 'Beta' was the standardized regression coefficient. 'Sig' was the significance level for the test of the null hypothesis that the value of a coefficient was zero in the population.

Estimation of Hockey Performance on the basis of selected physiological variables of Sub-Junior Hockey Players

Multiple Regression Analysis

The multiple regression equation for predicting the Hockey Performance on the basis of relative contribution of five physiological variables of sub-Junior group resulted in the following-

Equation-3

$$Y=16.430-0.037 (X_2) -0.031 (X_3) +0.005 (X_4) +0.043 (X_5) -0.398(X_6)$$

Y=Predictor (Hockey Performance)

X_2= Diastolic blood Pressure

X_3= Resting Heart Rate

X_4= Peak Flow Rate

X_5= Aerobic Capacity

X_6=Body Mass Index

The above mentioned regression equation shows that Hockey Performance depend upon the Diastolic blood Pressure, Resting Heart Rate, Peak Flow Rate, Aerobic Capacity and Body Mass Index.

Relationship between Hockey Performance and Physiological Variable of Sub-Junior Hockey Player are presented in Figure 27 to 32 and combined relationship between Hockey Performance and Selected Physiological Variable of Sub-Junior Hockey Player is shown in Figure 33.

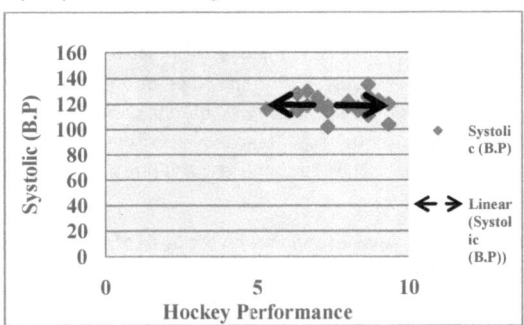

Figure-25: Relationship between Hockey Performance and Systolic (B.P) of Sub-Junior Hockey Players

83

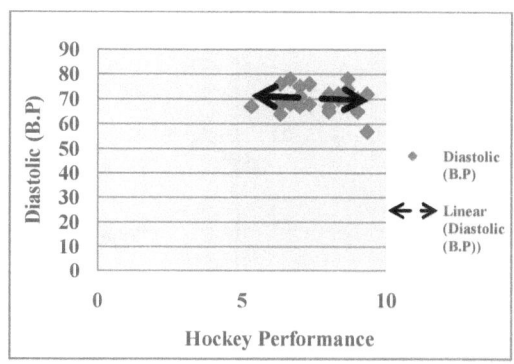

Figure-26: Relationship between Hockey Performance and Diastolic (B.P) of Sub-Junior Hockey Players

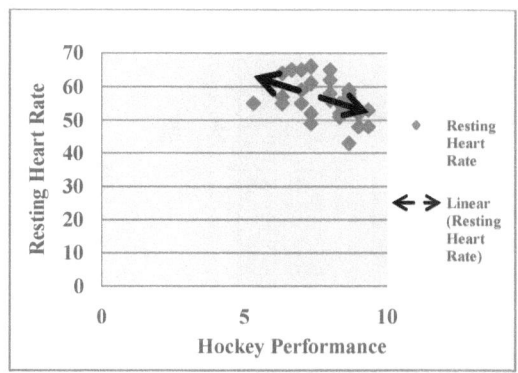

Figure-27: Relationship between Hockey Performance and Resting Heart Rate of Sub-Junior Hockey Players

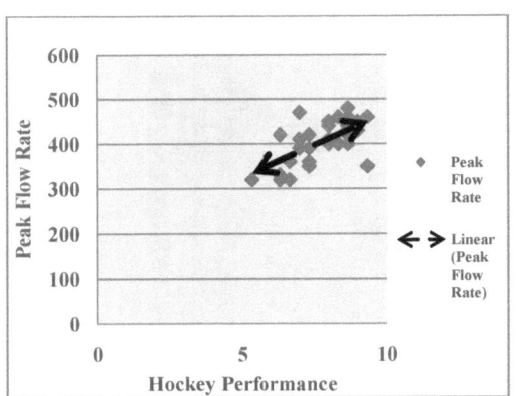

Figure-28: Relationship between Hockey Performance and Peak Flow Rate of Sub-Junior Hockey Players

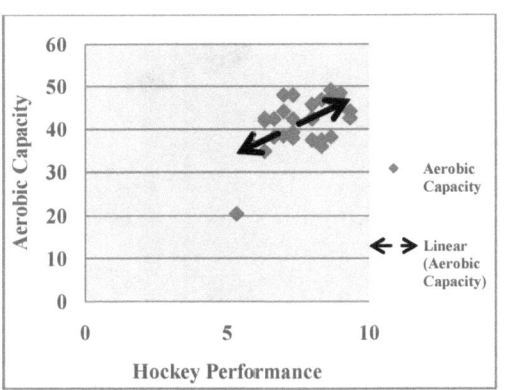

Figure-29: Relationship between Hockey Performance and Aerobic Capacity of Sub-Junior Hockey Players

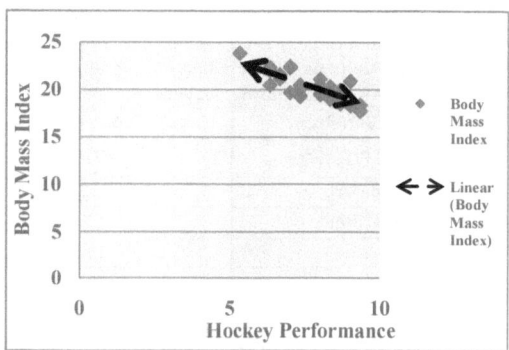

Figure-30: Relationship between Hockey Performance and Body Mass Index of Sub-Junior Hockey Players

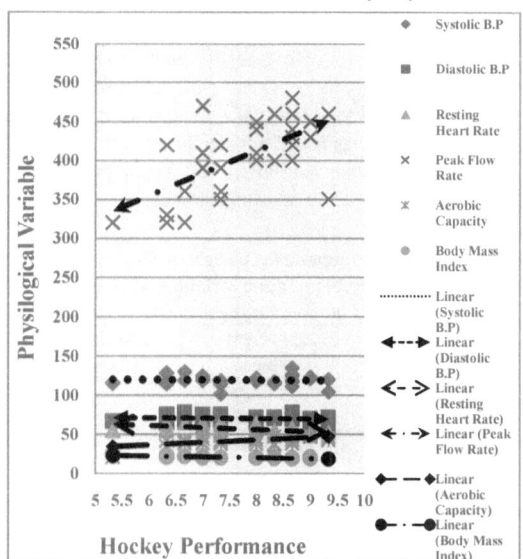

Figure-31: Combined Relationship between Dependent Variable (Hockey Performance) and Independent Variable (Selected Physiological Variable) of Sub- Junior Hockey Players

TABLE – 23

Relationship between Dependent Variable (Hockey Performance) and Independent Variables (Selected Physiological variables) of Junior Hockey Players

Independent Variables	Correlation coefficient
Systolic Blood Pressure	-.719*
Diastolic Blood Pressure	-.337
Resting Heart rate	-.531*
Peak flow rate	.551*
Aerobic capacity	.667*
Body mass index	-.640*

*Significant at .05 level

$r_{0.05}(28) = 0.361$

Table -20 revealed that Hockey performance was found significantly correlated with Systolic Blood Pressure, Resting Heart rate, Peak flow rate, Aerobic capacity, Body mass index as the correlation coefficient values (-.719, -.531, .551, .667, -.640) were found higher than the tabulated value at 0.05 level of significance. Hockey Performance was found not significant with Diastolic Blood Pressure as the correlation coefficient values were found lower than the tabulated value at 0.05 level of significance.

TABLE – 24

Joint Contribution of Independent Variables (Selected Physiological variables) in predicting Dependent Variable (Hockey Performance) of Junior Hockey Players

Criterion Variables	Independent variables	Coefficient of multiple correlation
Hockey Performance	Systolic Blood Pressure	0.876*
	Diastolic Blood Pressure	
	Resting Heart rate	
	Peak flow rate	
	Aerobic capacity	
	Body mass index	

* Significant at .05 level.

$r_{0.05}(23) = 0.396$

87

Table-21 indicates significant relationship between criterion variables *(Hockey Performance)* and independent variables (Selected Physiological Characteristics) as coefficient of multiple correlations was found 0.876 which is higher than the tabulated value.

TABLE – 25

Model Summary

R Square	Adjusted R Square	Standard Error
.767	.719	.684

The above table 22 shows that Adjusted R Square (.719) as predictor was included, which means that 71.9% of the variance in the performance of Hockey player was associated with changes in the physiological variable.

TABLE – 26

Analysis of Variance for the Regression

	Sum of Square	df	Mean Square	F	Significant
Regression	36.98	5	7.39		
Residual	11.23	24	.47	15.81*	.000
Total	48.20	29			

*Significant at .05 level

$F_{0.05}$ (5, 24) =2.51

Finding of table 23 revealed that developed regression model is significant for prediction of criterion variable and model can be used for further prediction, as value of 'F' (15.81) was found significant at 0.05 level of significance.

TABLE – 27

Coefficients[a]

Model	Unstandardized Coefficients		Standardized Coefficients	t	Sig.
	B	Std. Error	Beta		
(Constant)	30.915	5.789		5.341	.000
SYSTOLIC B. P RESTING	-.103	.031	-.482	- 3.285	.003
HEART RATE	-.080	.037	-.274	- 2.168	.040
PEAK FLOW RATE	-.011	.004	-.477	- 2.598	.016
AEROBIC CAPACITY	.120	.034	.545	3.549	.002
BODY MASS INDEX	-.271	.146	-.272	- 1.855	.076

a. Dependent Variable:

The above table displayed the value of the coefficient in the regression equation and measures the probability that a linear relationship existed between Physiological variables and the Hockey Performance. In this table 'B' was the slope of the line. 'SE B' was the standard error of 'B'. 'Beta' was the standardized regression coefficient. 'Sig' was the significance level for the test of the null hypothesis that the value of a coefficient was zero in the population.

Estimation of Hockey Performance on the basis of selected Physiological variables of Junior Hockey Players.

Multiple Regression Analysis

The multiple regression equation for predicting the Hockey Performance on the basis of relative contribution of five physiological variables of junior group resulted in the following-

Equation-4

$$Y = 30.915 - 0.103(X_1) - 0.080(X_3) - 0.011(X_4) + 0.120(X_5) - 0.271(X_6)$$

Y=Predictor (Hockey Performance)

X_1= Systolic blood Pressure

X_3= Resting Heart Rate

X_4= Peak Flow Rate

X_5= Aerobic Capacity

X_6=Body Mass Index

       The above mentioned regression equation shows that Hockey Performance depend upon the Systolic blood Pressure, Resting Heart Rate, Peak Flow Rate, Aerobic Capacity and Body Mass Index.

       Relationship between Hockey Performance and Physiological Variable of Junior Hockey Player are presented in Figure 34 to 39 and combined relationship between Hockey Performance and Selected Physiological Variable of Junior Hockey Player is shown in Figure 40.

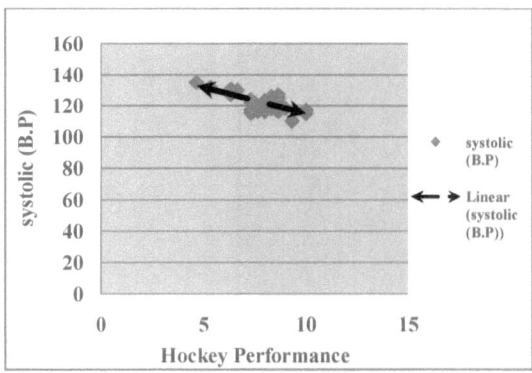

Figure-32: Relationship between Hockey Performance and systolic (B.P) of Junior Hockey Players

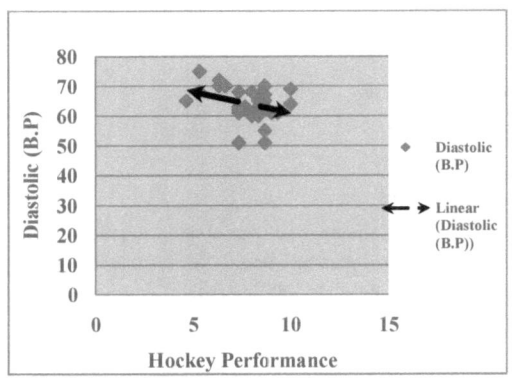

Figure-33: Relationship between Hockey Performance and Diastolic (B.P) of Junior Hockey Players

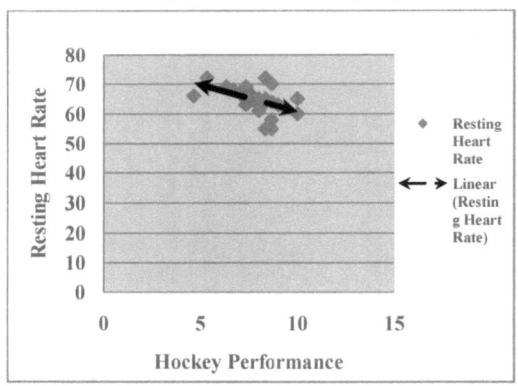

Figure-34: Relationship between Hockey Performance and Resting Heart Rateof Junior Hockey Players

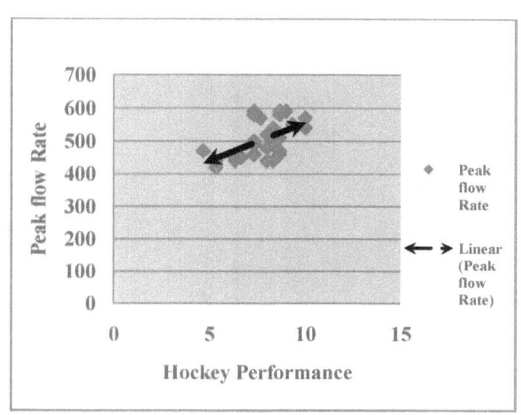

Figure-35: Relationship between Hockey Performance and Peak flow Rate of Junior Hockey Players

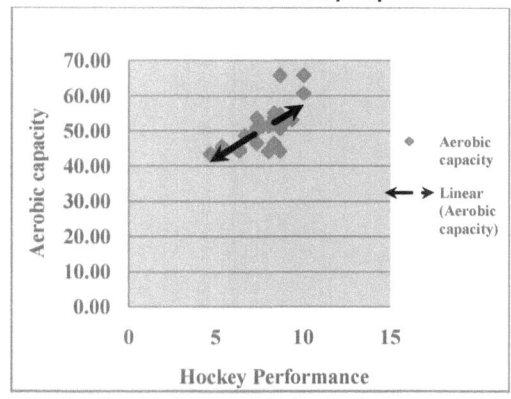

Figure-36: Relationship between Hockey Performance and Aerobic capacity of Junior Hockey Players

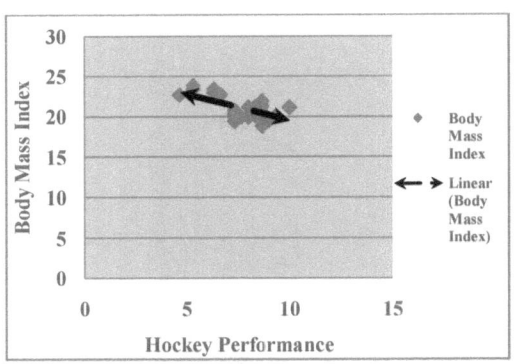

Figure-37: Relationship between Hockey Performance and Body
Mass Index of Junior Hockey Players

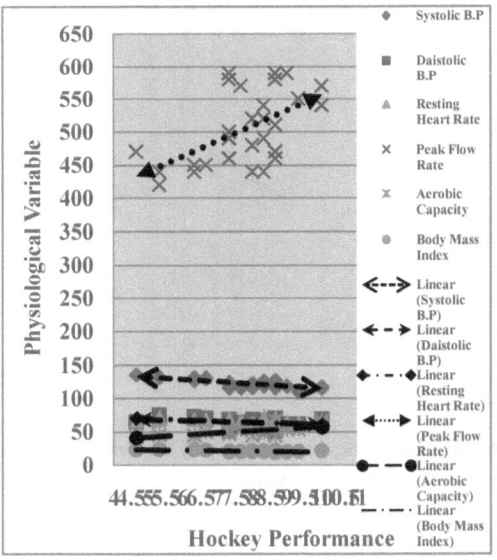

Figure-38: Combined Relationship between Dependent Variable
(Hockey Performance) and Independent Variable (Selected
Physiological Variable) of Junior Hockey Players

Discussion of findings

Research scholar had taken this study with a consideration that Anthropometric and physiological variables might have dominant and determinant role on performance of Sub-Junior and Junior Hockey players.

If the exact variable could be identified and which have most determinant predictive power for Hockey performance, it could be of immense training implication as well as tools/criteria for talent identification.

The findings of the statistical analysis have shown dominant role of selected variable for the Sub-Junior and Junior in terms of predictor of Hockey performance. Research scholar is of view that the findings have more than justified the purpose, for which the study was mainly taken up.

From anthropometric variables, weight and percentage of body fat were found to be significant in Hockey performance of Sub-Junior Hockey Players and weight and percentage of body fat were found to be significant in Hockey performance of Junior Hockey Players.

Similarly for Physiological variables, the primary determiners of Hockey performance, resting heart rate, peak flow rate, aerobic capacity, and body mass index were significant in Sub-Junior hockey performance while, systolic blood pressure, resting heart rate, peak flow rate, aerobic capacity and body mass index were significant in Junior hockey performance.

The statistical analysis of the data has clearly indicated that those selected anthropometric variables which were not significantly related to sub junior hockey performance i.e. height, arm length, leg length, and thigh girth. But in relation to multiple correlations, a significant multiple correlation coefficients were found between anthropometric variables and sub-junior hockey performance.

The statistical analysis of the data has clearly indicated that all selected anthropometric variables were not significantly related

94

to junior hockey performance i.e. height, arm length, leg length, thigh girth. But in relation to multiple correlations, a significant multiple correlation coefficients were found between anthropometric characteristics and junior hockey performance.

The monitoring and evaluation of such anthropometric variables, alongside game related performance characteristics, provides greater knowledge and understanding about the processes and consequences of selection, training and performance in youth sport (Till, et al., 2011). The findings of Sidhu J.S, (2013) who investigated the relationship between selected anthropometric variables of upper limbs (weight, height, sitting height, arm length, shoulder diameter, elbow diameter, chest circumferences, upper arm circumferences,) to the performance in male hockey players gave the similar conclusion that negative and non significant relationship exist between skin fold measurement (triceps, sub-scapula, suprailliac) to the performance in male hockey players. Results of the study Karkare A (2011) who investigated to compare anthropometric measurements and body composition of hockey players with respect to their playing position gave the similar conclusion that hockey players playing in different position found to differ on some anthropometric measurements and body composition.

The finding of the present study clearly revealed that anthropometric characteristics had a significant relationship with Hockey performance.

Results also revealed that the all selected physiological variables namely Resting Heart Rate, Peak Flow Rate, Aerobic Capacity and Body Mass Index are significantly related to sub-junior Hockey performance whereas systolic blood pressure, diastolic blood pressure are not significantly related to sub-junior Hockey performance. But in relation to multiple correlations, a significant multiple correlation coefficients were found between physiological variables and Hockey performance of sub-junior Hockey players.

Results also revealed that the all selected physiological variables namely Systolic Blood Pressure, Resting Heart Rate, Peak

Flow Rate, Aerobic Capacity and Body Mass Index are significantly related to junior Hockey performance whereas, diastolic blood pressure are not significantly related to junior Hockey performance. But in relation to multiple correlations, a significant multiple correlation coefficients were found between physiological variables and Hockey performance of junior Hockey players.

The reason for similarity of the result in both groups (junior and sub-junior) may be due to the fact that the players were of national level and reaching that level requires a very strenuous training for a long time. Results of Manna et al. (2010) who investigated the effect of training on selected anthropometric, physiological and biochemical variables of elite field hockey players gave the similar conclusion that no significant changes were noted in stature, body mass, HRmax, resting heart rate, VO2max and anaerobic power of the players after the training.. Results of the study conducted by Dutta (1984) on relationship of physical, physiological and psychological variable to performance in hockey gave the similar conclusion that significant relationship of hockey playing ability with speed, right grip strength, left grip strength, agility, balance, and a kinaesthetic perception, cardio respiratory endurance, resting pulse rate, hand reaction time, speed of movement, response time and body composition and anxiety but the relationship between standing broad jump, trunk flexibility and intelligence to hockey playing ability were not found to be statistically significant.

The finding of the present study clearly revealed that physiological variables had a significant relationship with Hockey performance.

Regression analysis employing Anthropometric and Physiological variables have shown distinctively different combinations of parameters, as Hockey performance determinate for Sub-junior and Junior Hockey Players.

Regression equation findings as shown above have mainly identified Height, Weight, Arm Length, Leg Length, Thigh Girth, Percentage of Body Fat from anthropometric characteristics and

Systolic Blood Pressure, Diastolic Blood Pressure, Resting Heart Rate, Peak Flow Rate, Aerobic Capacity, and Body Mass Index from Physiological variables, as a determining variables of Hockey performance National level of Sub-Junior and Junior Hockey Players.

In equation-1 the combination of height, weight, arm length, leg length, thigh girth, and percentage of body fat could provide a reasonably good estimation of hockey performance of sub-junior hockey player.

In equation-2 the combination of height, weight, arm length, leg length, and percentage of body fat could provide a reasonably good estimation of hockey performance of junior hockey player.

In equation-3 the combination of Diastolic blood Pressure, Resting Heart Rate, Peak Flow Rate, Aerobic Capacity and Body Mass Index could provide a reasonably good estimation of hockey performance of Sub-junior hockey player.

In equation-4 the combination of Systolic blood Pressure, Resting Heart Rate, Peak Flow Rate, Aerobic Capacity and Body Mass Index could provide a reasonably good estimation of hockey performance of junior hockey player.

Discussion of Hypothesis

In the light of the findings of the present study the hypothesis that there shall not be any significant relationship between dependent variable (Hockey performance) and independent variables (anthropometric and physiological variables), was not accepted in case of only two anthropometric variables i.e. Weight and percentage of body fat with Sub-Junior Hockey performance and with Junior Hockey performance. Also for Physiological variables i.e. Resting Heart Rate, Peak Flow Rate, Aerobic Capacity, Body Mass Index with Sub-Junior Hockey performance. Systolic blood pressure, Resting Heart Rate, Peak Flow Rate, Aerobic Capacity, Body Mass Index with Junior Hockey performance whereas accepted in case of all other selected Physiological variables i.e Systolic blood pressure and diastolic blood pressure with Sub-Junior Hockey performance and diastolic blood pressure with Junior Hockey performance and Anthropometric variables i.e height, arm length, leg length and thigh girth with Sub-Junior Hockey performance and height, arm length, leg length and thigh girth with Junior Hockey performance

But the second hypothesis that there shall not be any significant joint contribution of independent variables (selected anthropometric and physiological variables) in relation to dependent variable (Hockey performance) was not accepted in case of all selected Physiological variables and Anthropometric variables.

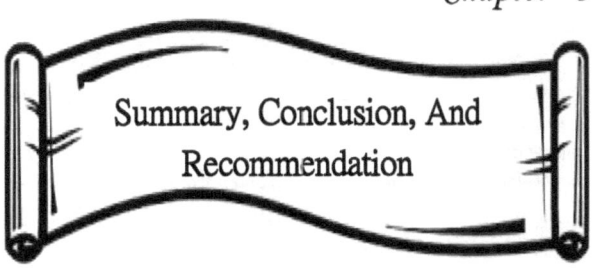

Chapter - 5

Summary, Conclusion, And Recommendation

Summary

The purpose of the study was to investigate the relationship of anthropometrical and physiological variables to performance of sub-junior and junior hockey players and to find out the combined contribution of anthropometric variables and physiological variables to performance of sub-junior and junior hockey players besides developing a multiple regression equation for the prediction of hockey performance of sub-junior and junior hockey players.

Sixty male Hockey players (thirty sub-juniors and thirty junior) were selected as subjects from National tournament. The dependent variable hockey performance and independent variable anthropometric and physiological variable. Hockey performance was determined by taking expert opinion from (out of 10 points) a panel of three experts and the average of three score was considered as hockey performance. Anthropometric variables included height, weight, arm length, leg length, thigh girth, percentage of body fat which was measured by Stadiometer, weighing machine, steel tape, skinfold calliper respectively. Physiological variables included blood pressure, resting heart rate, peak flow rate, aerobic capacity, body mass index were measured by digital blood pressure machine, heart beat per minute, peak flow mater, cooper's 12 minute run/walk test, the test were administered in hockey field of sports college of Lucknow and SAI centre Bhopal. For collection of data testers competency, subjects reliability, and reliability of tests were established by test- retest method and the reliability co-efficient were found to be satisfactorily high.

The data were analysed using the Pearson product moment (r) for assessing the relationship of the hockey performance to each of the anthropometric and physiological variables. Multiple correlation for assessing the combined contribution of anthropometric and physiological variables to performance and regression equation for predication the performance from anthropometric and physiological variables were applied. Level of significance for testing the null hypothesis was set at 0.05.

Analysis of data revealed significant relationship of performance of Sub-junior Hockey players anthropometric and physiological variables, weight (r=-.469), percentage of body fat (r=-.679), resting heart rate (r=-.463), peak flow rate (r=.621), aerobic capacity (r=.559), body mass index (r=-.783). The relationship between height, arm length, leg length, thigh girth, systolic blood pressure to performance Sub-junior Hockey players were not found to statistically significant at 0.05 level of confidence.

Analysis of data revealed significant relationship of performance of Junior Hockey players anthropometric and physiological variable, weight (r=-.453), percentage of body fat (r=-.796), systolic blood pressure (r=-.719), resting heart rate (r=-.531), peak flow rate (r=.551), aerobic capacity (r=.667), body mass index (r=-.640). The relationship between height, arm length, leg length, thigh girth, diastolic blood pressure to performance of Junior Hockey players were not found to statistically significant at 0.05 level of confidence.

Multiple correlation was computed to determine those anthropometric and physiological variables which contributed most to the hockey performance of sub-junior and junior hockey players. The result of the study indicated that the height (X1), weight (X2), arm length (X3), Leg length (X4), Thigh girth (X5), Percentage of body fat (X6) contribute most to sub- junior hockey performance with R= 0.914 among anthropometric variable, Diastolic blood pressure (X2), resting heart rate (X3), peak flow rate (X4), aerobic capacity (X5), body mass index (X6) contribute most to sub- junior hockey performance with R=0.891 among physiological variables.

Multiple correlation was also computed to determine those anthropometric and physiological variables which contributed most to the hockey performance of junior and junior hockey players. The result of the study indicated that the height (X1), weight (X2), arm length (X3), Leg length (X4), Percentage of body fat (X6) contribute most to junior hockey performance with R= 0.888 among anthropometric variable, systolic blood pressure (X2), resting heart rate (X3), peak flow rate (X4), aerobic capacity (X5), body mass index (X6) contribute most to junior hockey performance with R=0.876 among physiological variables.

Multiple regression analysis resulted in the following equation for anthropometric (A) and physiological (B) variables for sub junior hockey players:

A. $Y=8.103+0.344 (X_1) -0.236(X_2) -0.304(X_3)-0.071(X_4) +0.075(X_5) - 0.138 (X_6)$

B. $Y=16.430-0. 037 (X_2) -0.031 (X_3) +0. 005 (X_4) +0 .043 (X_5) - 0.398(X_6)$

Multiple regression analysis resulted in the following equation for anthropometric (A) and physiological (B) variables for junior hockey players:

(A) $Y=21.809+0.202 (X_1) -0.077 (X_2) -.327 (X_3)-0.129 (X_4) -0.442 (X_6)$

(B) $Y=30.915-0.103 (X_1) -0.080 (X_3) -0.011 (X_4) +0.120 (X_5) -0.271 (X_6)$

Conclusions

Within the limitation of the study, the following conclusions appeared justified as per the result obtains:

1. The Anthropometric variable namely weight and percentage of body fat are significantly related to performance of sub-junior hockey players.

2. Among physiological variables, resting heart rate, peak flow rate, aerobic capacity, and body mass index are significantly related to performance of sub-junior hockey players.

3. Height, arm length, leg length, and thigh girth (anthropometric variables) are not found significantly related to performance of sub-junior hockey players.

4. Systolic blood pressure and diastolic blood pressure (physiological variables) are not found significantly related to performance of sub-junior hockey players.

5. The Anthropometric variable namely weight and percentage of body fat are significantly related to performance of junior hockey players.

6. Among physiological variables systolic blood pressure, resting heart rate, peak flow rate, aerobic capacity, and body mass index are significantly related to performance of junior hockey players.

7. Height, arm length, leg length, and thigh girth (anthropometric variables) are not found to be significantly related to performance of junior hockey players.

8. Diastolic blood pressure (physiological variables) is not found to be significantly related to performance of junior hockey players.

9. Height, weight, arm length, Leg length, thigh girth and Percentage of body fat contribute most to sub- junior hockey performance.

10. The regression equation for estimating Hockey performance of sub-Junior Hockey players on the basis of selected Anthropometric variables is:

a. $Y=8.103+0.344$ (X1) $-0.236(X2)$ $-0.304(X3)-0.071(X4)+0.075(X5)-0.138(X6)$

11. Diastolic blood pressure, resting heart rate, peak flow rate, aerobic capacity and, body mass index contribute most to sub-junior Hockey performance.

12. The regression equation for estimating Hockey performance of sub-Junior Hockey players on the basis of selected Physiological variables is:

a. $Y=16.430-0.037 (X_2) -0.031 (X_3) +0.005 (X_4) +0.043 (X_5) - 0.398(X_6)$

13. Height, weight, arm length, Leg length, and Percentage of body fat contribute most to junior Hockey performance.

14. 16. The regression equation for estimating Hockey performance of Junior Hockey players on the basis of selected Anthropometric *variables* is:

a. $Y=21.809+0.202 (X_1) -0.077 (X_2) -.327 (X_3)-0.129 (X_4) -0.442 (X_6)$

15. Systolic blood pressure, resting heart rate, peak flow rate, aerobic capacity and, body mass index contribute most to junior Hockey performance.

16. The regression equation for estimating Hockey performance of sub-Junior Hockey players on the basis of selected Physiological variables is:

a. $Y=30.915-0.103 (X_1) -0.080 (X_3) -0.011 (X_4) +0.120 (X_5) -0.271 (X_6)$

Recommendation

In light of the result of this study, it is recommended that:

1. The results of the study can be used by the physical education teachers and coaches as an aid in screening and selecting prospective Sub- Junior and junior hockey players.

2. Since the anthropometric and Physiological variables have greater relevance to the performance in hockey game, influence of measurements of different parts of body other than those employed in the study and their effects on performance may be a worthy area of study.

3. It is recommended that similar study may be repeated by selecting subjects belonging to age groups and level of achievements other than those employed in the present study.

4. The similar study of nature can be conducted on female players of different level of achievement.

5. It is recommended that similar study may be conducted by using Physical and psychological variables.

6. The study may be undertaken with large number of variables

7. Similar study may be under taken to analyze the other games players and athletes.

8. This study can be conducted on International teams.

9. Similar study may be conducted on senior Hockey Players.

BIBLIOGRAPHY

Books

1. Balke, Burno (1979) *"Variation in Altitude and Its Effect on Exercise Performance"*, cited by Harold B Falls Exercise Physiology, New York: Academic Press.

2. Barry L. Johnson, Jack K. Nelson (1982), *"Practical Measurement for Evaluation in Physical education"* Surjeet Publication, Delhi.

3. Best J.W (1963) *"Research in Education"*, U.S.A.: Prentice Hall.

4. Buchar C.A. (1975) *"Foundation of Physical Education"*, St. Louis: The C. V. Mosby Company.

5. Clark, H. H., & Clark, D. H. (1975) *"Research Process in Physical Education"* Englewood cliffs, New Jersey: Prentice Hall, Inc.

6. Dirix A, Knuttgen H.P, Title K (1988), *"The Olympic Book of Sports Medicine"*, Vol. 1 of the Encyclopedia of Sports Publication in Collaboration with the International Alteration of Sports Medicine.

7. Donald K. Mathews (1978), *"Measurement in Physical Education"*, 5th ed. Philadelphia: W.B, Saunder, Co.

8. Dubey H.C. (1999) *"Hockey"* Discovery publishing house, New Delhi.

9. Dureha D.K, Mehrotra A (2003), *"Teaching and Coaching Hockey"*, Janvani Prakashan (p) Ltd., Delhi.

10. Gay, L.R. (2000) *"Educational Research"*, U.S.A: Prentice Hall.

11. Harre, *"Principles of Sports Training"*.

12. Kansal D. K (1996) *"Test and Measurement in Sports and Physical Education"*, New Delhi, D.V.S. Publication.

13. Lawry G. Shaver (1981), *"Essentials of Exercise Physiology"* Surjeet Publication, Delhi.

14. Matveyev L (1981) *"Fundamentals of Sports Training"*, Moscow Progress Publishers.

15. McGrath, Charles (2008), "*A Chinese Hinterland, Fertile With Field Hockey*", New York Times.

16. Morehouse, Laurance E, Miller, Augustus T (1967) *"Physiology of Exercise"*, 7th ed. Saint Louis, C.V. Mosby company.

17. Pheasant S (1996) *"Body Space: Anthropometry, Ergonomics and Design of Work"*, Taylor & Francis, New York.

18. Philips A, Harnok J. E (1979) *"Measurement and Evaluation in Physical Education"*, New York: John Willey & Sons.

19. Prakash, Verma J (2000) *"A Text Book on Sports Statistics"*, Gwalior: Venus Publication.

20. Robert, V. *"Hockey Practical Fitness: The Path-Way of Healthful Living"*, St. Louis: the C.V Mosby Company.

21. Singh S. P, Malhotra P (1989) *"Kinanthropometric"*, Lunar Publications, Malhotra Textiles, Chowk Fort, Patiala.

22. Sodhi M.S, Sodhi L.S (1984) *"Physique and Selection of Sports Person"*, Punjab publishing house, Patiala.

23. Sodhi, H. S. (1991) *"Sports Anthopometry"* Anova Publication, Mohali.

24. Taylor, Vear (1988), *"Taylor on Hockey"* (Queen Anne press, Macdonald & Co (Publishers) Ltd., 3rd floor, Great Britain).

25. Werner, W.K., Hoeger, Sharon, A. Hoeger (1990), *"Fitness and Wellness,"* (USA: Morton Publishing Company).

Journals and Periodical

1. Atkinson G, Nevill A.M. (2001) "Selected Issues in the Design and Analysis of Sport Performance Research", *Journal of Sports Sciences*, Vol. 19, 811-827

2. Chauhan M.S. (2006) "Correlation between Selected Anthropometric Variables and Middle Distance Running Performance", *Sports Authority of India*, NSNIS Patiala.

3. Chauhan M.S, Sehgal, Subash., Yadav D (2009) "Prediction of Sprinting Ability of Secondary School Boys of Haryana in Relation to their Anthropometric Measurements." *Sports Authority of India*, NSNIS Patiala.

4. Diwarka (1991) "Selected Physical, Physiological and Motor Skill Determinants of Performance in Female Inter-College Level Volleyball Players of Himachal State.

5. Dravin, Singh Y, Bangari D (2013) "Comparative Investigation of Anthropometric Physical Fitness and Skill Measurements of Selected Hockey Players of Uttar Pradesh" *International Journal of Behavioural Social and Movement Sciences,* Vol.02, Issue 01.

6. Elferink-Gemser, M.T., Visscher, C., Lemmink K.A., and Mulder T.W, (2004). "Relation between Multidimensional Performance Characteristics and Level of Performance in Talented Youth Field Hockey Players" *Journal of Sports Sciences*, Vol. 22, 1053-1063.

7. Elferink-Gemser, M.T., Visscher, C., Lemmink, K.A.P.M., and Mulder, (2007). "Multidimensional Performance Characteristics and Performance Level in Talented Youth Field Hockey Players: A Longitudinal Study" *Journal of Sports Sciences* (Pending Minor Revisions).

8. Francise. Holway, Marianoseara (2011) "Kinanthropometry of World Champion Junior Male Field Hockey Players" *Apunts Medicine Esport.*

9. Gabbett, T.J. (2000) "Physiological and Anthropometric Characteristics of Amateur Rugby League Players", *British Journal of Sports Medicine*, Vol. 34(4), 303-307.

10. Gil, S.M., J. Gil, F. Ruiz, A. Irazusta, and J. Irazusta (2007) "Physiological and Anthropometric Characteristics of Young Soccer Players according to Their Playing Position: Relevance for the Selection Process", *Journal of strength and conditioning research*: the research journal of the NSCA, Vol. 21, 438-445.

11. Gravina, L., Gil, S.M., Ruiz, F., Zubero, J., Gil, J.,& Irazusta, J. (2008) "Anthropometric and Physiological differences between First Team and Reserve Soccer Players aged 10-14

Years at the beginning and End of the Season", *Journal of Strength and Conditioning Research*, Vol. 22(4), 1308-1314.

12. Hughes M.D, Barlett M (2002) "The Use of Performance Indicators in Performance Analysis", *Journal of Sports Sciences,* Vol. 20, 739-754.

13. Indranil Manna, Gulshan Lal Khanna , Prakash Chandra Dhara (2010) "Effect of Training on Anthropometric, Physiological and Biochemical Variables of Elite Field Hockey Players" *International Journal of Sports Science and Engineering* Vol. 04(4), 229-238

14. Jusice M. Boseworth (1965), "Relationship Between the Vertical Jump Performance of College Women and Selected Anthropometric Measurements and Strength Variable," *Completed Research in Health, Physical Education and Recreation.* Vol.7: 93.

15. Stagno K.M, Thatcher R., Someren K.A. Van (2005) "Seasonal Variation in The Physiological Profile of High level Male Field Hockey Players" *Biology of Sport*, Vol. 22 No. 2

16. Karkare A. (2011) "Anthropometric Measurements and Body Composition of Hockey Players with Respect to their Playing Positions", *Indian Streams Research Journal*, Vol.1:5-8.

17. Keogh, Justin W.L, Weber, Clare L, Dalton, Carl T (2003) "Evaluation Of Anthropometric, Physiological, and Skill-Related Tests for Talent Identification in Female Field Hockey" *Canadian Journal Of Applied Physiology*, Vol. 28 (3), 397.

18. Khanna, G. L, Majumdar P, Malik V, Vrinda T, Mandal M (1996) "A Study of Physiological Responses during Match Play in Indian National Kabaddi Players", *British Journal of Sports Medicine,* Vol. 30(3), 232-235.

19. Malhotra M.S, Joseph N.T, Mathur D.N, Gupta S J (1975) "Physiological Assessment of India Hockey Players", *Sports Medicine*, Vol. 2: 5 -10.

20. Manna I, Khanna G, Dhara P (2009) "Training Induced Changes on Physiological and Biochemical Variables of Young Indian Field Hockey Players", *Biology of Sport*. Vol. 26(1):33-43.

21. Manna I, Khanna G. L, Dhara P. C *(2010)* "Study of Selected Physiological and Health Related Variables of Indian Field Hockey Players of Different Age Groups Following A Pre-Competition Training" *Asian Journal of Exercise and Sports Science,* Vol. 7 No 1.

22. Randal W. Reid, (1978) "The Relationship of Lower Limb Flexibility, Strength and Anthropometric Measures to Skating Speed in Varsity Hockey Players" *Completed Research in Hearth, Physical Education and Recreation* Vol. 20: 144.

23. Reilly, T, Bretherton S (1986) "Multivariate Analysis of Fitness of Female Field Hockey Players", In Perspectives in kinanthropometry (edited by J.A.P. Day), *Human Kinetics*, pp. 135-142

24. Reilly T, Borrie A (1942) "Physiology Applied to Field Hockey", *Sports Medicine,* Vol.14:10-26

25. Reilly T, Seaton A (1990) "Physiological Strain Unique to Field Hockey" The *Journal of Sports Medicine and Physical Fitness*, Vol. 30, 142-146.

26. Sangral M.S (1984), "Motor Fitness Components as Predictor of Talent in Hockey". *Indian Journal of Sports Sciences and Physical Fitness*, Vol. 6:52.

27. Sidhu J.S. (2013) "Relationship of Selected Anthropometric Variables of Upper Limbs to the Performance in Male Hockey Players", *Futuristic Trends in Physical Education,* Vol. 1: 94-98

28. Singh M, Singh M.K, Singh K. (2010) "Anthropometric Measurements, Body Composition and Physical Parameters of Indian, Pakistani and Sri Lankan Field Hockey Players", *Serbian Journal of Sports Sciences,* Vol. 4(2): 47-52.

29. Starkes, J.L. (1993) "Skill in Field Hockey: The nature of the cognitive advantage", *Journal of Sport Psychology,* Vol. 9, 146-160

30. Reilly T, Bangsbo J and Franks A (2000), "Anthropometric and Physiological Predispositions for Elite Soccer" *Journal of Sports Sciences*, Vol. 18, 669-683.

31. Tarverdizadeh, B, Azarbayjani, M.A. (2012) "Relationship of Anthropometric with Physical and Motor Fitness Features in Iranian Elite Soccer Players". *International Journal of Health, Physical Education and Computer Science in Sports:* Vol. 5(1), 16-17.

32. Throsen A, Margaret (1964) "Body Structure and Design Factors in the Motor Performance of College Women", *Research Quarterly* Vol. 35, 418.

33. Till, K, Cobley S, O'Hara J, Brightmore A, Cooke C, Chapman C (2011) "Using Anthropometric and Performance Characteristics to Predict Selection in Junior UK Rugby League Players", *Journal of Science and Medicine in Sport,* Vol.14(3), 264-269.

34. Van R, J.H.A. (2000) "Deliberate practice and Dutch field hockey: An addendum to Starkes", *International Journal of Sport Psychology*, Vol. 31, 452-460.

35. Viswanathan J, Chandrasekaran K (2011) "Optimizing Position-wise Anthropometric Models for Prediction of Playing Ability among Elite Indian Basketball Players" *International Journal of Sports Science and Engineering* Vol. 05(2), 067-076

36. Wassmer D J, Mookerjee S, (2002) "A Descriptive Profile of Elite U.S. Women's Collegiate Field Hockey Players", Vol. 42(2):165-71

37. Weber, C. L, Keogh J. C. L. (2000) "Physiological and Skill Based Characteristics in Female Senior and Junior Field Hockey Players" Pre-Olympic Congress Sports Medicine and Physical Education, *International Congress on Sport Science*, p. 7-13

Unpublished Thesis

1. Dureha D. K (1984) "*Comparison of Selected Motor Components and Anthropometric Variables of Offensive and*

Defensive College level Hockey Players" (Unpublished Master's Thesis, Jiwaji University, Gwalior).

2. Dutta A. K. (1984) *"Investigation of Selected Physical, Physiological and Psychological Assessment as Predictive Factor in Hockey Performance"* (Unpublished Doctor of Philosophy thesis, LNCPE Jiwaji University Gwalior).

3. Lamba M.K, (1980) *"Comparative study of selected Physical Fitness components and Physiological Parameters of Offensive and Defensive Hockey Players of College Level"* (Unpublished Master's Thesis, Jiwaji University, Gwalior).

4. Mohamed A (1997)*"Anthropometric Characteristics and Physiological Performance Variables of Male and Female Junior Hockey Players in Kwazulu Natal"* (Unpublished Master's Thesis, Department Of Physiology University Of Natal, Medical School, Durban).

5. Sidhu J.S (2012) *"Prediction of Performance of University Hockey Players in Relation to their Anthropometric and Physical Fitness Variables"*. (Unpublished Doctoral Thesis, Punjabi University, Patiala)

6. Vaz L. W. (1994) *"Investigation of selected anthropometric characteristics and physical fitness components as predictors of performance in judo."* (Unpublished Doctoral Thesis, Jiwaji University, Gwalior).

Miscellaneous

1. Durnin J.V.G.A, Rahman N.M. (1967) "Percentage of body fat corresponding to the total value of skinfold" *British Journal of Nutrition* 21:681.

2. Norton K, Olds T, Olive S, Craig N. (1996) Anthropometry and sports performance in Norton K Olds T ,editors *.Anthropometrical,* Sydney, Australia: University of New South Wales Press;.

3. Ross W. D, Ward R, Leahy R. M, Day J. A. P. (1982) Proportionality of Mon- treal athletes. In: Carter JEL, editor, The physical structure of athletes, Part I: *The Montreal*

Olympic Games Anthropological Project. Basel, Switzerland: Karger; .p.81—106.

4. Throsen A. Margaret (1964), "Body Structure and Design Factors in the Motor Performance of College Women", *Research Quarterly,* 35, 418.

http://www.ncbi.nlm.nih.gov/pubmed/12956036

www.Answer.com

www.google.com

www.pubmed.com

www.medterms.com

www.wikipedia.com